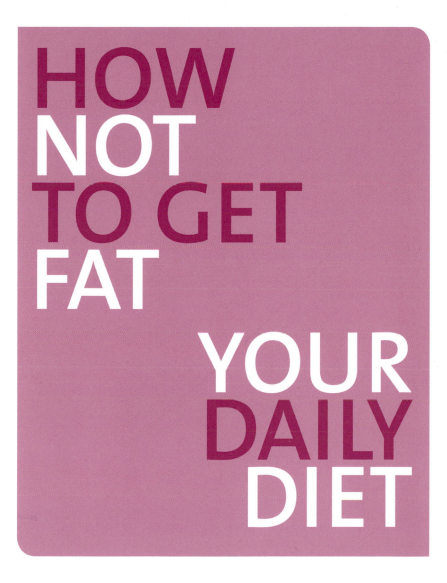

HOW NOT TO GET FAT YOUR DAILY DIET

Quadrille
PUBLISHING

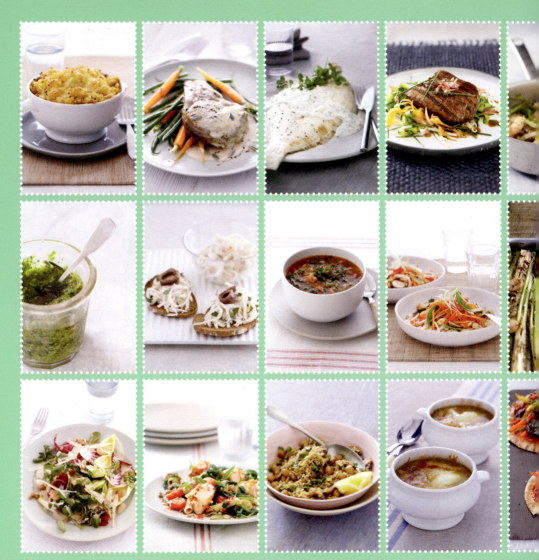

IAN MARBER

RECIPES BY CAROLYN HUMPHRIES

HOW NOT TO GET FAT
YOUR DAILY DIET

For Tim, my brother-in-law, and Jack, my nephew

First published in 2010 by
Quadrille Publishing Limited
Alhambra House
27–31 Charing Cross Road
London WC2H OLS

Editorial Director Jane O'Shea
Creative Director Helen Lewis
Editor Susannah Steel
Design and Art Direction Gabriella Le Grazie
Photography Rob Streeter
Food Styling Lucy McKelvie
Props Styling Wei Tang
Production Vincent Smith, Ruth Deary

Cataloguing in Publication Data: a catalogue record for this book is
available from the British Library.

ISBN 978 184400 934 3

Printed in China

Contents

Introduction

Hopefully you ate breakfast this morning. Even if you didn't give it much thought, you made a decision about what you wanted to eat. Perhaps you ate cereal or toast, drank fruit juice, and had a tea or a coffee. You may have chosen wholemeal toast or wholegrain cereal, organic fruit juice, and fairtrade tea or coffee with low-fat skimmed milk. On the surface, these are all quite respectable and entirely understandable choices. The juice is a good source of vitamin C and the cereal might be rich in minerals and vitamins – which perhaps influenced your decisions. So it may come as a surprise to know that, despite the healthy implications of your choices, they could be making you gain weight over time.

We are more informed about nutrition than ever before, yet in the West we are generally becoming fatter. I believe that this is because nutrition and weight management have become confused and the concept of 'healthy eating' is now an increasingly muddled term. The truth is that even nutrient-rich foods can cause weight gain. The fact that fruit juice contains vitamin C and cereal offers minerals and vitamins is not of primary relevance when it comes to managing weight; when learning how to eat in a way that manages their weight, not one of my clients has ever discussed with me whether particular foods contain a certain vitamin or mineral. If you make food choices solely due to nutritional content, then these good intentions highlight just how many of us are eating what we think is a good diet, but one that can still result in slow but steady weight gain. For example, choosing low-fat processed foods in an effort to reduce your calorie intake often leads to you eating more sugar, which leads to fluctuations in levels of blood glucose – something we will look at over the coming pages.

So if you are among the millions of people who have happened to gain weight, what now? Obviously you should go on a diet and lose weight, shouldn't you? But which diet? Think of the diets that have been popular over the last ten years. We have seen them come and go, and maybe you have tried some of them. Most of them work – for a while, at least – until we eat normally again, when the weight returns. And the next time it's harder to lose the weight, isn't it?

Perhaps you feel that you have no weight issues and you can eat what you like without putting on weight. Or perhaps you may not be carrying any extra weight because you eat carefully and exercise regularly. But have you ever read about some amazing diet plan that seems so easy and allows you to eat anything you like? Have you tried it, just in case, because you can always lose five pounds and it would be nice to be just that little bit leaner? Even the most grounded of people can be forgiven for doing this: over the years, the diets that have been most popular are those that claim to have discovered a basic scientific principle that has previously been overlooked. Needless to say, this concept is immensely attractive to us, not least because the media inevitably debates its merits and that only increases its popularity.

It is the repeated cycle of dieting that I believe is one of the primary reasons why we are getting fatter. Being 'on a diet' forces the body to consider that it is experiencing a famine, and, over time, it adapts to manage the new calorie intake. As soon as we complete the diet and return to eating normally (albeit an improved version of what we were eating before dieting), our body will store away additional calories in readiness for the next famine. Sure enough, there will be another famine, as we want to lose the weight again. So the cycle continues until we end up larger than we ever imagined we could be.

Of course, it's hard to relate to extremes – to people who are so large they have to have walls cut down in order to leave the house – but these obese people weren't born fat. They grew fat, and then fatter still. Instead, you might be the sort of person who loses weight in January, only to gain it all back again in time to lose it for the summer holidays. You then lose weight in preparation for Christmas when you pile it back on again. Perhaps it's harder to lose weight the second or third time, so you have to diet a little harder or exercise just that little bit more to shift the pounds. This day-to-day dieting doesn't attract much media attention, so it is considered almost normal: a news headline such as 'Woman Loses Weight after Christmas' will never catch our eye in the same way that 'Man has to be Winched out of Bed' might.

If you relate to this day-to-day dieting scenario, then you, too, are a seasoned dieter. Some people seem destined to spend the rest of their lives either on or off a diet, feeling 'good' or being 'bad'. Given the choice between eating in a way that makes you gain and lose weight repeatedly over the years, or enjoying varied foods that prevent weight gain, I think it's obvious which you might choose. Prevention simply has to be better than cure. But for the majority of us in the West, we don't even know that there is such a choice. We have been exposed to a lifetime of advertising, marketing, and media interest in diets, so it's understandable that we tend to follow the 'boom or bust' or 'feast or famine' pattern of eating.

So here's the good news: there is another way to eat – one that enables you to manage your weight, promotes energy, reduces hunger, and still provides all the good nutrition that you might require – and that's what this book is about. *Your Daily Diet* is the middle ground that allows us to eat, not diet: to enjoy food without having to use willpower to control ourselves. I know that this plan does what it says, not just because it works personally for me but because I have spent many years developing, perfecting, tweaking, and refining it by learning from the experience of several thousands of my clients who have followed it. In this book I'll show you how to follow it so that you, too, can become immune to dieting.

In my last book, *How Not To Get Fat*, we explored some simple biochemistry showing how foods are converted into either energy or fat. We also looked at the influence of the media, and how many of us eat in a way that is totally at odds with how the body works. In this book the simple science and our lifestyles come together:

you will know exactly what to eat and when to eat it. If that sounds like a diet, then please be assured that it is not. It is straightforward, you don't get hungry, it supplies all the nutrition you need, and you can eat this way for the rest of your life.

In section one we'll remind ourselves of the basic facts involved in making energy from what we eat and drink, and I'll show you how to eat in a way that is in harmony with the way your body works. You won't be made to feel guilty and you won't have to learn how to compensate for overeating by undereating. On this plan you will be eating plenty of wholesome, nutritious food – not diet products.

Section two provides information on which foods fall into which food group, so you can be clear about whether a food is a protein or a complex carbohydrate. All you have to do is choose one food from each food group and combine them to make a snack or meal. There is plenty of advice about each food and simple suggestions for cooking and serving it. You don't be have to be a competent cook, or even that confident in the kitchen, as these pages explain how to put together a quick snack or a main course using basic ingredients. There are also some new and exciting recipes to try.

Finally, in section three we will meet a few fictional characters that represent many of us at various ages and stages, what they typically eat, and the mistakes they make. I have devised meal plans for each character to show how they can change their eating habits for the better. Pick the scenario you identify with most and use the meal plan as a blueprint for your own daily diet.

I know that *Your Daily Diet* will show you how to eat well in a way that maximises your energy levels while ensuring that you don't gain weight, which should spare you a lifetime of dieting.

Ian

www.thefooddoctor.com

Section one

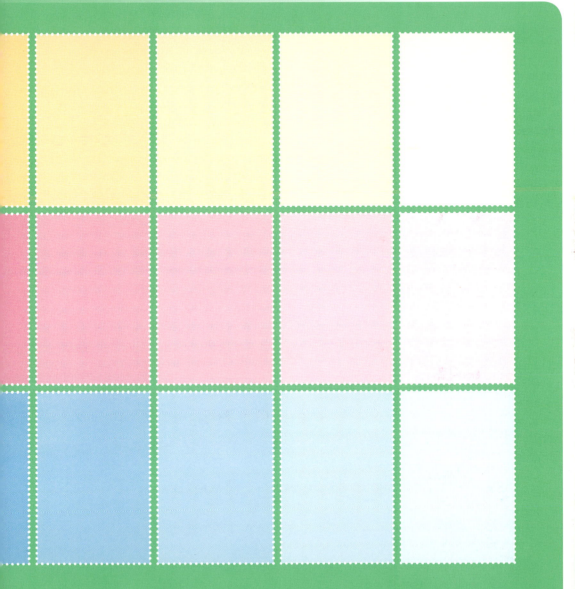

How food becomes energy

The basic science I learned at school didn't teach me much about human nutrition, and it wasn't until I studied nutrition when I was in my thirties that I realised how little I actually knew about what I was eating.

Things are different these days, as nutrition and diet are in the forefront of many people's minds. There is perhaps almost too much information, which has led to confusion and even inappropriate eating, along with fad diets and increased levels of obesity. Confusion can be avoided if we learn some simple facts about how the human body works.

It's important that we understand some basic science and, even if you have read my previous book, *How Not To Get Fat*, I suggest you still read this section so that you are comfortable with the concepts of my plan.

Why do we eat?

Of course, there are many answers to this question. Food is associated with satisfaction, pleasure, conviviality, and numerous other factors, but essentially we eat in order to survive. We need food to create the energy required by every cell, muscle, tissue, enzyme, organ, and bone in our bodies to function properly – and we often overlook this fact as we battle with food. When it comes to our growing children, we have no problem feeding them if they are hungry and need energy. But as adults the urge to eat has become tainted with so many issues that we often forget that food provides that essential fuel we need to keep going.

We are affected by what we eat and drink, and that influences our appetite and energy. *How Not To Get Fat* looks at the physiological issues involved in eating and how they impact our psychology – in other words, how we work and how we behave as a result of what we eat.

So a quick reminder about how food becomes energy is appropriate here to highlight some of aspects of this process that we can influence for the better. Bear in mind that the processes we are about to explore are happening right now in your body.

Turning food into fuel

The transformation of a mouthful of food into fuel occurs in the digestive system, and that process starts in the mouth. The aim of chewing our food is to turn the food into a soft pulp so we can swallow it. As we chew, the food mixes with our saliva, which contains weak enzymes that begin to break down the bonds that hold the food together. Next stop is the stomach, where hydrochloric acid repeatedly washes over the food, further breaking down the various bonds in it. Although this acid is fairly powerful, we need to ensure that we chew our food well so that when it enters the stomach, it is in a suitable state for the acid to work most effectively.

The presence of food in the stomach triggers the release into the bloodstream of three hormones – which are directly involved with appetite: gastric inhibitory peptide (GIP), cholecystokinin (CCK), and secretin. GIP and CCK are generally triggered only by the presence of fat in food, although protein will trigger some, too. They automatically send a signal to the brain to tell us that we have had enough food.

This is the moment to mention another hormone, leptin, which is also linked to reducing appetite, and which has been found to be at its highest level after eating fish, beans, and fresh produce (we'll return to leptin, CCK, and GIP again later).

When the stomach is ready to release its contents – now a viscous liquid – it is pushed into the upper section of the gut. As this thick liquid moves through the rest of the digestive system, glucose and nutrients are extracted from it and absorbed through the lining of the intestine into the bloodstream.

Glucose

Glucose is derived from food and distributed around the body in the bloodstream to cells that can use it to create energy. Glucose is a vital aspect of how not to get fat, so it's really important to make sure that you are familiar with what glucose does, and how to manage it.

Having been a nutrition therapist for 12 years now, it's true to say that I have described and explained glucose management many times every working day. Each time I do so I am reminded of just how crucial this aspect of weight control really is. So please read on, even if you are familiar with this topic

Glucose must lurk around cells waiting to enter; the cell is a sealed unit and won't absorb glucose until tiny channels in its perimeter are opened up. Once these channels are open, they allow the glucose to seep slowly into the cell where the biochemical processes can get to work and convert it into energy.

A simple formula for glucose:
Glucose enters a cell and, once inside, it passes through several biochemical processes and is converted into energy

Glucose and insulin (a hormone that regulates the amount of glucose in the blood) form the cornerstone of how the human body uses food to create energy. This simple equation (below) underlines the importance of glucose and insulin and their relationship to each other.

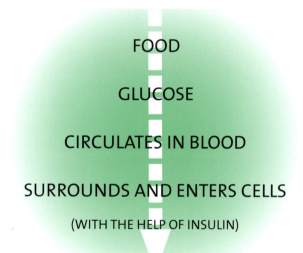

FOOD

GLUCOSE

CIRCULATES IN BLOOD

SURROUNDS AND ENTERS CELLS

(WITH THE HELP OF INSULIN)

Over the years, I have used a few analogies to describe glucose management. One that seems to work well is of traffic: if you think of glucose as vehicles and insulin as the traffic police, this may help to make the issue of glucose management easier to relate to

Glucose management

Large amounts of glucose in the blood lead to a traffic jam as the vehicles try and get into the cells. All this time, still more glucose is continuing to join the bottleneck (in other words, as glucose waits to gain entry to a cell, more glucose crowds around it because more of the food you recently ate has been broken down).

The cell is closed off from the rest of its environment by a barrier, and in order for 'vehicles' to gain access to the cell the barrier has to be opened. The barrier stays firmly closed until the signal to open is received, and that signal comes from insulin. Insulin levels in the blood are low when glucose levels are low. As glucose levels start to build, so does insulin. Traffic police are dispatched to deal with traffic jams, so I hope this is an easy analogy to imagine.

Once the cells get the signal to open the barrier, glucose can get into them. Remember that the channels allowing glucose in are limited, so even though the cells are now open, not much glucose can flow in at any one time. In terms of traffic, the roads that lead out of the traffic jam are narrow, and even if they are accessible, the vehicles have to wait patiently until it's their turn to go.

Insulin manages glucose in two ways: first by signalling the cells to enable them to open; and secondly by removing the excess glucose and sending it to fat cells for storage. In terms of vehicles, those that are waiting to get in line for the single file traffic heading for the cells are diverted from the traffic jam and sent down another route.

There is one more important point to make here. As new glucose enters the bloodstream, if it encounters insulin early on it can be sent straight to storage rather than even getting as far as waiting in line to enter a cell. Using the traffic analogy again, new vehicles encountering the roads that are jammed up ahead will be directed away rather than allowing them to join the traffic jam.

So, to summarise:
- ▸ Food is broken down into glucose in the digestive system
- ▸ Glucose is transported all over the body in the bloodstream
- ▸ Insulin signals the cells to allow glucose in
- ▸ The glucose that is excess to requirements is stored in fat cells

Food groups

We now need to take a look at food and understand a little about how much glucose different foods create.

The foods that we eat can be divided into three basic groups:

- ‣ Carbohydrates
- ‣ Protein
- ‣ Fats

These can be divided further into subgroups:

- ‣ Carbohydrates: simple and complex
- ‣ Proteins: complete and incomplete
- ‣ Fats: essential and non-essential

For our purposes we are going to focus on the three basic groups, but include both simple and complex carbohydrates, as the subgroups of proteins and fats are not so relevant here (although there is some more information on them in the introduction to section 2). Examples of what kinds of foods fall into the three groups are listed in the table (opposite).

If you take a look at the list below, you will see how the food groups are ranked according to the speed at which they are broken down by the digestive system:

1st   Simple carbohydrates
2nd   Complex carbohydrates
3rd   Proteins
4th   Fats

Examples of foods in the three basic groups (including the two subgroups of carbohydrates)

SIMPLE CARBOHYDRATES (4 calories per gram)	COMPLEX CARBOHYDRATES (4 calories per gram)	PROTEINS (4 calories per gram)	FATS (9 calories per gram)
Sugar	Green and salad vegetables	Meat	Dairy products
Cereals (most)	Beans	Poultry	Fish
Jam	Firm fruit	Fish	Seeds
Cakes	Grapefruit	Nuts	Red meat
Biscuits	Brown rice	Seeds	Poultry
Pasta made with white flour	Pasta made with wholewheat flour	Soya and soy products (such as tofu)	Oils (such as olive oil)
White bread	Oats	Quinoa	Nuts
Dried fruit	Brown bread	Quorn	
Fruit juice	Barley	Beans	
Milk	Rye		

It is interesting to note, looking at the calorie content of each food group in brackets at the top of each column, that fat contains the greatest amount of calories. If you were to follow a diet that concentrates solely on limiting calories, you would aim to eat as little fat as possible, as it is so high in calories (low-fat diets may automatically be lower in calories). However, as we have already seen, dietary fats contribute to the pleasing sensation of eating, trigger hormones that signal the brain to get us to stop eating (p.13), and are very slow to break down in the body.

So in spite of its higher calorie score, eating fat has benefits that seem to outweigh this disadvantage

Digesting the different food groups

The physical form of various foods is obviously different, some being dense and hard to chew (such as a carrot), others requiring comparatively little chewing (such as a grape), and some that don't need chewing at all (such as carrot juice). Fat is especially hard to break down by the body because it has a relatively complicated structure, while carbohydrates are far easier for the body to digest. For example, a slice of soft white bread, which is a simple carbohydrate (see box, p.17), requires very little chewing and so is easy for the body to convert into glucose. Not only is it easy to break down the bonds in the white bread, the process of extracting glucose from a simple carbohydrate such as this doesn't take long. So eating a slice of white bread will create a fair amount of glucose in the bloodstream quite quickly.

As we know that excess glucose leads to increased fat stores, would one piece of white bread lead to weight gain? The answer is 'no': just one slice won't create much glucose, even if it is created so quickly. The amount of glucose derived from the bread is still at a level that the cells can absorb without allowing any glucose to be stored away. But what would happen if you ate two slices of white bread? At this point the glucose levels are likely to become too concentrated, which means that insulin will grab the excess glucose to store it away (in other words, there is now too much traffic on the road so the police must direct some away from the bottleneck).

If you had just one slice of white bread, but added some strawberry jam to it, what would happen then? Strawberry jam is made from cooked fruit and sugar, both simple carbohydrates. Like the bread eaten on its own, a glut of glucose would ensue from this combination of foods, only this time there would again be too much glucose, which leads to glucose being stored as fat (and therefore probable weight gain).

So we know that simple carbohydrates eaten on their own or with other simple carbohydrates provide the body with a rush of glucose. What happens if you eat a food from another food group, such as protein? A small, grilled chicken fillet, for example, requires plenty of chewing until it is in a comfortable state to swallow. Once in the stomach, the hydrochloric acid has to work hard to break the food down, partly because of its physical structure, but also because proteins actually take longer to make glucose when they are absorbed. So eating a chicken breast will create glucose in a slow and consistent way that doesn't flood the cell. Thinking again in terms of the traffic analogy, eating a protein creates traffic in single file that all moves in an orderly fashion and therefore escapes the attention of the traffic police.

And what about fat? A slice of cheese is primarily a fat, but it also contains protein. Fats get broken down into two elements: fatty acids, which make up the majority of the fats that we eat, and glycerol. Only glycerol is converted into glucose. So the body takes time to create glucose, of which there isn't much anyway. So of the three foods, cheese has the lowest impact on the concentration of glucose in the blood.

There are two things to be aware of with fat:
▸ Eating fat creates texture in the mouth that provides a feeling of satisfaction and pleasure, which enhances the experience of eating.
▸ Eating fat triggers various hormones to be released (leptin, CCK, and GIP), which tell the brain that we are full, so we eat less.

How do I feel?

Until now I have focused on the physiological aspects of how glucose levels in the blood rise and fall, but how does this corresponding fluctuation in energy levels make us feel, and how does it affect our food choices?

We know that food is broken down to create glucose, which is fed into the cells to create energy. So the ebb and flow of glucose levels in the blood link directly to whether we feel energised or fatigued. It would follow that plenty of glucose would equal plenty of energy, right? Well, only partially right, and certainly only in the short term. This is because eating a meal or a snack that is rapidly converted into glucose supplies the cells with fuel – but the glucose that can't be absorbed is sent away for storage. Insulin is responsible for this and acts in a random manner, sweeping away as much glucose as it can.

What insulin doesn't do is leave glucose in the blood for later, in case you need more energy. It has no idea you ate a big breakfast to see you through the morning, nor does it care if you are trying to lose weight. Insulin does its job of managing glucose levels consistently; it never varies in its regulatory role

As I mentioned, you might think that plenty of glucose in the blood would amount to plenty of energy, but this is only partially true. As insulin responds to high levels of glucose in the blood by indiscriminately grabbing whatever glucose it can as soon as it hits the bloodstream, the amount of glucose available to enter the cell is still limited.

In other words, the amount of glucose that creates enough energy is only that glucose which is in the right place at the right time

Remember that glucose is always circulating in the blood, and whenever there is glucose, insulin is present, too. If the levels of both glucose and insulin were tested immediately on waking without you having eaten, their levels would be low and in proportion, but they would change as soon as you ate or drank something.

So, if eating a food creates a glut of glucose, some of which is stored away, do you feel energised or fatigued immediately after this process has occurred? Obviously you won't be aware that it's happening, so perhaps you might not make the connection between what you ate for breakfast and how tired you feel by the time you get to work (or your children get to school). But we do experience rises and falls in glucose levels, as you will see. And how does what you feel influence your choices as to what you eat next? A low in glucose levels leads to a low in energy levels, something that you experience as hunger. We know that when a baby cries or a child is grumpy, the chances are that they are hungry and we respond accordingly. When the same hunger occurs in an adult or teenager, however, the response is often not quite so straightforward.

What influences our food choices?

From a very young age we are exposed to food advertising and marketing on television, on billboards, and with celebrity representation (sometimes taking the form of a cartoon character). More recently the marketing of products has evolved into social networking sites, online games, and communities targeting every user, especially the young.

In order to understand how profoundly we are all influenced by marketing and advertising, let's create a mythical breakfast cereal, 'Corn Rice Honeyed Puffs', and follow its journey from the field to a young child's body

Corn and rice are low-cost grains and the honey may be of commercial quality (which also translates into a lower cost). The grains are puffed, which fills them with air and reduces their fibre content. Even after factoring in manufacturing and packaging costs, the cereal provides a high profit margin for the manufacturer, providing it with funds to spend on advertising and marketing. The manufacturer might pay a license fee to an animated filmmaker to use characters from his newest film production, or he might create a cartoon character of his own. The use of the names of the basic ingredients – corn, rice, and honey – in the title implies that they are 'good' foods: rice comes from a field and therefore is natural, as is corn, and honey is from bees, which equates to 'nature', so the cereal implies that it should also be 'good' for us. The recipe also contains very little fat, so the maker can correctly claim that it is low in fat, something that is highlighted on the front of the pack.

We have seen that eating carbohydrates can lead to a glut of glucose, especially processed foods that fall into the simple carbohydrate category. And as there is little or no fat or protein in the Corn Rice Honeyed Puffs to slow down the process of digestion, eating our cereal leads to a level of glucose in the blood that is too concentrated. In turn, this triggers increasing levels of insulin to deal with it (or a holiday weekend's worth of traffic trying to get through a bottleneck, causing the traffic police to arrive to deal with the chaos).

But all that's of little interest to a young child who has experienced everything associated with the cereal in the media. This might include a character or image that personalises the cereal being featured on billboards, television, and online. And once the cereal is a commercial success, the manufacturer might extend the successful brand into cereal snack bars using the same colours, images, slogans, and advertising campaigns. Back to our child: it's Saturday morning, a couple of hours have passed since breakfast, and he is hungry. The family is out shopping and the parents, knowing their son is hungry, offer him the choice of an apple or a cereal bar as a snack.

The cereal bar obviously has more appeal to the boy, as he is familiar with Corn Rice Honeyed Puff cereal bars from the various promotions (apple growers are unlikely to spend much on advertising or marketing, as apples have little profit margin, which makes the apple far less prominent in the child's psyche). The boy's parents may prefer that their son has an apple, but as the bar boasts that it is low in fat and contains corn and rice they buy it. So the child eats the snack bar and the glucose levels in his blood rise rapidly, causing his insulin levels to rise in tandem.

This rapid rise of glucose levels in the young boy can be attributed to three aspects of the Corn Rice Honeyed Puff cereal bar:
1. It contains honey
2. It has little or no fat or protein in it
3. The grains have been processed to shape them, which has removed the majority of their inherent fibre

The glucose that does enter cells creates energy, but the rest is swept away and stored, eventually being added to the fat cells. The boy experiences this process only as a short-term boost in energy (so, returning to the analogy, once the vehicles at the head of the queue have been directed through the bottleneck, those waiting further back have been directed away and what is left is mostly an empty road). The energy created by eating the snack bar is only short-lived, leading the boy to feel tired and hungry again within a short space of time.

    If you wouldn't dream of letting a child have sugared treats, and would offer dried fruits or an organic cereal bar instead, don't be fooled. These foods might not generate the same concentrated levels of glucose and insulin in the body, which in turn quickly lead to fatigue and hunger, but they still create more glucose in the bloodstream than the cells can absorb in a short period of time. Expand this example of eating a snack bar to a whole day's eating and you can see how the hunger that comes with this way of eating increases along with our waistlines.

Putting the theory into practice
We know from the example of the cereal bar made from our mythical Corn Rice Honeyed Puffs that eating a sweetened, processed grain leads to glucose highs, and we also know how that affects our energy levels. Let's apply this knowledge to two foods from the other food groups and track the response both physiologically and psychologically.

Peanuts
Like all nuts, peanuts contain both protein and fat and are also dense and fibrous. This combination challenges the digestive system to the extent that extracting the glucose from the nuts takes a long time; the glucose is extracted slowly and consistently. Therefore, the first dose of glucose that enters the bloodstream is limited. In turn, this triggers just enough insulin into the blood to signal to the cells to absorb circulating glucose, but not enough insulin to sweep away the excess, as there isn't any.

At nine calories per gram, it takes about 20 peanuts (a heaped palmful) to equal the calorie count of our imaginary cereal bar. But the calories from the nuts do not cause a spike in insulin levels; the glucose drip-feeds into the cells slowly and consistently. Only once that glucose has run out do we feel hungry again.

Had the boy in our scenario eaten peanuts instead of the bar, he would have felt well-fed and satisfied for longer than he did

Eating fat and protein alone, however, is not advised, simply because it leads to an acid environment in the body, as well as having a potentially negative effect on blood lipids such as cholesterol. We don't need to linger too much on this point, but when we eat too much protein the body becomes acidic, taking the pH level a little too low. We weren't built for this, so the body cleverly compensates for this by making the environment more alkaline to even things out, and in doing so it dips into its reserves of minerals, mainly calcium. In the long term this can lead to a reduction in bone density, while the short-term repercussions can include constipation and muscle cramps. There is also evidence that a long-term acid environment in the body can increase the incidence of some forms of cancer.

A slice of wholegrain bread

Unlike the white bread I mentioned earlier (p.18), wholegrain bread is a complex carbohydrate (p.17) made from brown flour that has not been milled to the same degree as white flour. Its higher fibre content is harder for the digestive system to break down and extract glucose from.

However, wholegrain bread is still a carbohydrate that, even when digested, and unlike proteins and fats, is converted easily into glucose. Remember that the process of digestion is faster for carbohydrates, as is the conversion into glucose – a double whammy, if you will.

Wholegrain bread is considered 'better' than white bread, but eaten alone it, too, will lead to a glucose glut, an insulin spike, short-term energy, and potential weight gain. The fact that there is an inferior alternative in the form of white bread, a simple carbohydrate, has made us feel rather kindly towards complex carbohydrates, but in my opinion they are not good when eaten alone.

Why combine the food groups?

Let's put these two different foods together – the slice of wholegrain bread spread with some peanuts ground into a crunchy peanut butter (the type sold in every supermarket, but without sugar). This combination of the food groups creates the ideal amount of glucose in the blood, leading to short- and medium-term energy.

Although there are even more calories in eating a slice of wholegrain bread with peanut butter than eating them separately, together these foods take even longer to digest and the energy they create lasts longer.

This is a vital concept in my eating plan, and Your Daily Diet depends upon it: always eat protein and complex carbohydrates together

Never eat just protein and never eat just complex carbohydrates, but always, without fail, eat them together. If this sounds too technical or hard to follow, it's not. Think of a typical lunch you might buy when you are out and about or at work. A sandwich is an obvious choice, and if it contains a protein such as chicken, and maybe lettuce and tomato, it is a complete meal – protein with complex carbohydrates (salad vegetables and bread) and a little fat (from the chicken). Just make sure that there is enough protein and the bread is wholemeal or wholegrain.

The number of combinations really is endless. Section two includes a huge selection of meal and snack recipes to inspire you, and in section three I will show you how to tailor your meals and snacks to suit your personal tastes and preferences.

By combining the food groups correctly, you take care of several aspects of eating:

- Balance between alkaline and acid
- Excellent levels of fibre
- Reduced hunger
- Consistent energy levels
- Consistent glucose levels
- Rich in nutrients

No weight gain

So how do we add the requirement of no weight gain to this impressive list? The answer is easy: eat every two and a half to three hours, starting every day with breakfast. If you eat a combination of the food groups and ensure that your portion size is not too large, the amount of glucose created should last you for two and a half to three hours. By eating this regularly through your waking hours, you will have a consistent level of energy. Typically, this means eating the following meals in a day:

- Breakfast
- A mid-morning snack
- Lunch
- An afternoon snack
- Dinner

However, I know from many of readers of *How Not To Get Fat* who have successfully gained control of their diets by eating this way, that there are sometimes occasions when they need a further snack. This might be between the afternoon snack and a late dinner, or a small snack later in the evening after an early dinner.

So there are two important guidelines to this plan:
1. Combine the food groups
2. Eat every two and a half to three hours

Daytime and evening

There is, however, one more important point to note: you need the right ratio of protein to carbohydrates during the day, and a slightly different one in the evenings. The reason may be obvious: from breakfast onwards we are likely to be active and busy with work, family, and living our lives, but in the evenings the chances are that you aren't so active. Also, at night (unless you work nights) you need less immediate glucose until the morning, when you are up and around again.

Therefore for dinner and an evening snack, if you have one, you should combine protein with complex carbohydrates derived from green and salad vegetables only.

The different complex carbohydrates

There is a subtle difference between the complex carbohydrates derived from fruits and vegetables and those derived from grains (sometimes called starchy carbohydrates).

I don't want to oversimplify this but, in general, most vegetables contain small amounts of the carbohydrates that influence blood glucose, whereas grain-based carbohydrates contain much larger amounts. It is true that some vegetables do influence glucose levels more than others, but if we start listing those that are good, not so good, and to be avoided, I think that constitutes a diet, doesn't it? There is one simple fact here that means you don't have to worry about which vegetables, fruit, or grain you choose to eat: any carbohydrate eaten with a protein will have significantly less negative impact on blood glucose level than when eaten on its own. I hope this helps to explain again why I believe in this mantra:

It is imperative that we always eat protein with complex carbohydrates. Always. Without fail. Every single time

A word about breakfast

Eating something within 30 to 60 minutes of waking up in the morning is a must. I know of many yo-yo dieters who choose to eat breakfast at work, so they eat something at around 9.30 a.m. after having already been up for two hours. As keeping your glucose levels consistent is an integral part of this plan, it is imperative that you eat something within an hour of waking. If you don't have much of an appetite in the mornings – and I appreciate that some people may not – then have a banana and a palmful of almonds, or an apple and a small slice of hard cheese, or a cold hard-boiled egg and two oatcakes. As long as you have a combination of the food groups, this will work. You can still have breakfast when you get to the office, but only eat a small portion, as you will soon be having a snack in the middle of the morning.

Exercise or activity?

Needless to say, exercise is an integral part of weight management, but I don't hold with the notion that you have to exercise intensively to 'burn off calories'. The truth is that of course you do have to exercise, but in order to maintain a healthy weight, or even lose weight, the trick is to be consistent. I can think of numerous clients who felt that they were fit because they went to the gym twice a week, but in truth those two one-hour sessions were the only physical activity they undertook during that week. They hardly walked anywhere and weren't involved in a sport, so despite the time spent in the gym, I doubt that they were that fit.

By all means continue with your weekly visits to the gym, but aim to do some sort of activity almost every day – and certainly not less than five times a week – for at least 30 minutes per day. Above all, involve yourself in physical activities that bring you some pleasure and satisfaction. Exercising this way brings so many health benefits that the investment of time and energy in it always pays off.

So now apply this knowledge to your own daily diet.

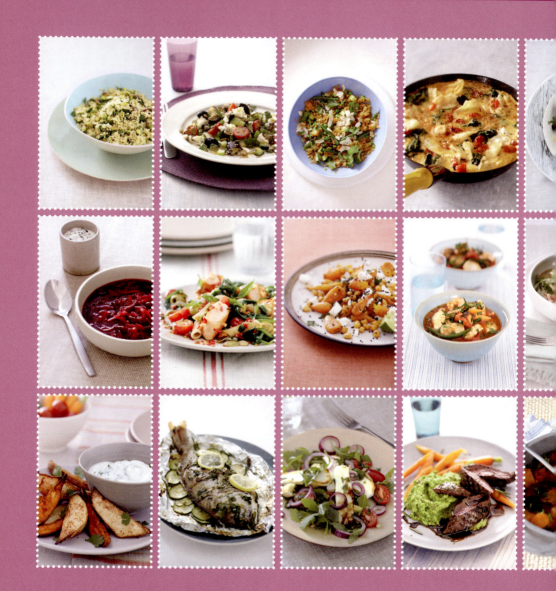

Section two

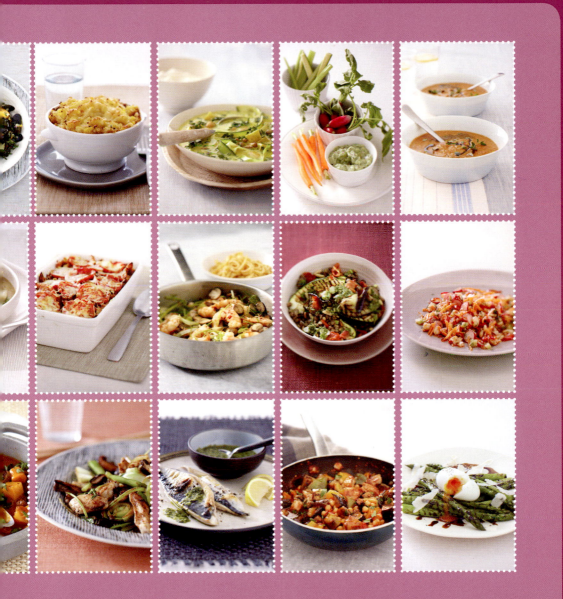

50 foods to eat

Introduction

I hope that you are now familiar with the three food groups, protein, carbohydrates, and fat. Most foods fall neatly into one of these three groups – although nearly all foods will contain a little of all of them. They each have a multitude of roles to perform in the body, ranging from a source of fuel to providing the building blocks for growth and repair. For our purposes, all we need to know is that they are broken down into glucose at differing speeds, which we can use to our advantage by combining them in a specific ratio by eating at regular intervals.

I feel it's important to eat different foods rather than face the same menu every day, which can be dull and uninspiring. So on the following pages you can read about 50 familiar foods, understand which category they fall into, and find out how to include them in your diet. Simply choose a carbohydrate and match it with a protein. You will see plenty of examples throughout this section of how to put together a meal or snack, and there are delicious recipes to try, but in essence you could flick through this section to a carbohydrate and combine it with a randomly chosen protein. You might end up with an odd combination, but if that's what you want, go ahead and enjoy it.

Complete and incomplete proteins

Proteins are an important part of a good diet, but not all proteins are created the same: some sources of protein will do the job just fine, while others need to be mixed with another protein to keep you feeling fuller for longer.

Proteins contain amino acids, eight of which are required by the body as 'building blocks'. The body can't generate these amino acids itself, but it can break them down and reconfigure them to make 14 more amino acids. If a protein contains all eight essential amino acids, it is considered a 'complete' protein, whereas one that doesn't is deemed to be 'incomplete'.

The rule of thumb is that proteins derived from animal sources such as red meat, poultry, eggs, fish, and dairy produce are complete proteins. Vegetable-based proteins are often incomplete, although there are some exceptions such as soy, spirulina, and quinoa. In the context of this daily plan it doesn't make a significant difference if you eat a protein that is complete or incomplete, so long as you don't eat incomplete proteins on their own all the time. As beans or legumes are nearly all incomplete proteins, just combine them with another legume or bean, or another protein such as poultry or fish, as together they will inevitably contain the ideal range of 22 amino acids.

Canned and frozen vegetables

Frozen vegetables are a very good standby, and in some cases they can be as nutritious as fresh produce, so keep a few packets of vegetables in the freezer.

Canned vegetables are also worth keeping in the store-cupboard, as long as the water they are stored in is unsalted and without sugar. Canned vegetables are not quite as nutritious as fresh or frozen produce, as the heating process can reduce their water-soluble nutrients, but I don't think this is especially significant if they are only eaten now and again.

Organic food

I am often asked about organic food and whether it is a requirement of a healthy eating plan. In the realms of *Your Daily Diet*, organic produce is not essential to success, simply because our focus is on combining the food groups and eating very regularly. Having said that, however, there are some health benefits, as yet largely unproven, to eating food that has been grown with minimal chemicals and antibiotics. The choice is always a personal one, but solely in this context, organic food is not necessary.

What to drink

What you drink is an essential part of this plan, and once again the focus is on how it influences glucose in the blood and not on its calorie content. Typically, we drink water, tea, coffee, juices, alcohol, and carbonated soft drinks. With the exception of water, all these drinks will probably have an impact on glucose levels. Caffeine mimics the effects of stress and encourages the body to produce adrenaline, which increases glucose levels. Alcohol, especially beer and wine, behaves like a simple carbohydrate that increases glucose levels. Fruit juices have had all their fibre removed and so act like a simple carbohydrates too. Carbonated soft drinks contain either sugar or caffeine, and often both. What we need to drink for the majority of the time should be free of caffeine, sugar, and simple carbohydrates. Water satisfies all these criteria, but here are some tips about other drinks:

• Drink tea and coffee with food – never in place of it, or first thing in the morning without eating anything – to minimise their influence on your glucose levels. Herbal tea contains no caffeine and can be enjoyed all day. Green and white tea both contain a little caffeine, but with levels low enough to make them suitable for all-day drinking. Decaffeinated tea and coffee are also acceptable, as they have little impact on glucose levels.

• Treat juice as part of the carbohydrate element of your meal. So have a glass of juice in place of fresh fruit with your yoghurt or cereal at breakfast. You still need to add a protein, so add flaked almonds or similar to the yoghurt. Bear in mind that if you have juice with tea or coffee, this will cause glucose levels to rise. So you need to choose one or the other.

• Carbonated soft drinks should be avoided unless they are completely free of caffeine and sugar. Although they may have several other health implications, artificial sweeteners do work as part of this plan, as they are sugar-free.

Sugar and chocolate

As sugar is the simplest of simple carbohydrates, it is turned into glucose very easily and, even if eaten with other foods, will lead to excess glucose levels. Avoiding sugar both on its own and as an ingredient in other foods greatly reduces the impact of this, making your hunger and your energy levels easier to manage. Eating sweet foods also tends to increase cravings for more of them. So rather than rely upon willpower, avoid sugar in the first place. Check the ingredients labels on foods; sugar can crop up in unlikely places.

Chocolate obviously contains sugar, so strictly speaking you shouldn't eat it. However, if you want to have some chocolate I suggest eating a few squares of very dark chocolate with a cocoa content of 80 per cent – and only eat this type – every now and again. Milk chocolate and chocolate that claims to be dark, but has a cocoa content of less than 80 per cent, don't qualify. If you want to eat chocolate, try a couple of squares with a few grapes to satisfy a sweet tooth, or add a few plain nuts that count as your protein for a snack.

Fruit

Despite its other health benefits, fruit should be eaten in moderation on this plan and your vegetable intake should increase in its place, as the fructose (fruit sugar) that fruit contains will affect your overall glucose levels. The speed at which a particular fruit affects glucose levels depends on how sweet it is and its fibre content. For example, papaya is relatively sweet to taste and is quite soft (with low/medium levels of fibre); this combination means that it has a medium-fast affect on glucose levels. Pineapple is far sweeter, but it also more fibrous, so it has a similar effect as papaya, since the fibre balances the sweetness. The best fruits to choose are those that have a low fruit sugar content and are fibrous; apples are a typical example.

Fruits are classified as a carbohydrate, so they should be eaten with a protein to ensure an even release of glucose. Be aware that fruit eaten at the end of a full meal can promote the fermentation of food in the stomach, which contributes to bloating and affects good digestion. So eating fruit as a dessert should be an occasional treat. You can enjoy many whole fruits without being overly concerned about which particular fruits to eat. All these fruits are suitable (fruit is best eaten fresh):

Apples	Grapes
Apricots (fresh)	Mangoes
Bananas	Papaya
Berries (blackberries, blueberries, loganberries, etc)	Peaches
	Pears
Cherries	Pineapples
Citrus fruits (lemons, limes, oranges, tangerines)	Plums
	Strawberries
Grapefruit	

Chicken and turkey

These meats are versatile proteins and good alternatives to red meat, as they generally contain less fat. The skin, however, does contain significant amounts of saturated fat and is unnecessarily high in calories, so remove it before eating. The white breast meat of chicken and turkey is the most popular and tender cut, but the dark leg or thigh meat is just as nutritious, full of flavour, and cheaper. Both marry well with numerous different flavours and ingredients, and can be cooked in a variety of quick, simple ways.

Choose birds with firm, plump flesh and milky-white, tight skin that look and smell fresh. Corn-fed chicken will have yellow skin and a rich flavour. If buying turkey steaks or chicken fillets, they should be moist, but not wet.

Sugar (as well as salt, water, and preservatives) is often added to pre-cooked poultry products so be aware that it may be present in the meat and sometimes on the skin, too. If the recipe ingredients list sugar, avoid these products.

Three simple cooking techniques

Stir-fry (or sauté) Heat 1–2 tablespoons of oil in a wok or large frying pan. Stir-fry diced or strips of poultry or chicken livers for 3–5 minutes until cooked through. If combining with stir-fry vegetables, add these after 2 minutes. Flavour with soy sauce, ginger, etc, as desired. For flattened steaks or breasts (escalopes), season and then sauté for about 3 minutes each side; for whole breasts or portions, 12–20 minutes, turning two or three times.

Poach Place a whole bird or pieces of meat in a saucepan. Cover with water or chicken stock. Add other flavourings as required (such as a bay leaf and an onion). Bring to the boil, reduce the heat, cover, and simmer very gently for 10 minutes for breasts or diced poultry, and 1 hour for a whole medium bird. If you prefer, leave the whole bird or plain poached pieces to cool in the liquid and serve the meat cold. Use the cooking stock as a soup base.

Stew or casserole Brown the meat quickly in a little oil with a chopped onion in a flameproof casserole or large saucepan. Add some vegetables, seasoning, herbs or other flavourings, and cover with chopped tomatoes and/or chicken stock. Bring to the boil, cover, then either reduce the heat and simmer very gently or transfer to the oven at 180°C (Gas 4) for 1 hour or until tender.

Meal suggestions

▶ Roast chicken or turkey with a selection of roasted root vegetables, some leafy greens, and gravy made with the meat juices and some chicken stock boiled until reduced then seasoned. Or serve with a crisp salad with a dressing of lemon juice and oil (for lunch, add new or jacket potatoes).

▶ Grilled chicken breast or turkey steak (flavoured as described, right) with the cooking juices poured over it and served with steamed vegetables (for lunch, add couscous).

▶ Chicken thighs stewed or casseroled in canned, chopped tomatoes with a handful of black olives thrown in and served with a green salad (for lunch, add mixed brown and wild rice).

▶ Grilled minced turkey or chicken burgers (pure meat, seasoned, bound with beaten egg, shaped into burgers, then brushed with oil) with a salad of bean sprouts, avocado, cherry tomatoes, and celery (for lunch, add wholegrain rolls).

▶ Warm chicken liver salad: trim the livers, season, and stir-fry (left). Pile onto bistro salad leaves (baby leaves with some shredded raw beetroot). Pour a little balsamic vinegar and olive oil into the pan, swirl round, and drizzle over the meat. Add a good grinding of black pepper and serve (for lunch, add warm new potatoes or multigrain bread).

Snack suggestions

▶ 2 slices of leftover roast chicken or a drumstick with crudités

▶ Chopped leftover roast chicken or turkey with 1/2 a sliced avocado in 1 wholemeal pitta bread

▶ Chicken liver pâté on 2 wholemeal crackers or 1 piece of wholemeal toast, with a few slices of cucumber

▶ Cold chopped chicken or turkey meat mixed into a small portion of leftover rice with some chopped salad vegetables and a handful of pumpkin seeds, moistened with a little French dressing

▶ Open turkey sandwich on a slice of wholemeal bread with some chopped celery, walnuts, and apple (all mixed with a little mayonnaise) spooned on top

What to look for
• Chicken: sold fresh or frozen as a whole bird, quarter portions (wing and breast, or leg and thigh), breasts with or without bone, thighs, wings, drumsticks, diced breast or thigh meat, mince, chicken livers (chicken wings and legs tend to have little meat on them once the skin is removed)
• Turkey: whole bird (fresh mostly at Christmas and Easter), steak and breast fillets, diced breast and thigh meat, wings, legs, and mince

Ways to cook or serve
• Boil
• Roast
• Grill
• Stir-fry or sauté
• Poach
• Stew or casserole

Simple ways to flavour
• Flavoured oil or pesto (p.80); smear over the meat before grilling or roasting
• Herbs (chopped fresh or dried): basil, oregano, parsley, rosemary, sage, tarragon, thyme
• Spices: cumin, chilli, curry pastes, paprika
• Tomatoes, onions, leeks, mushrooms, olives, and garlic

Chicken, shiitake mushroom, and pak choi stir-fry

You can use turkey or pork stir-fry meat instead of chicken for this dish if you prefer, and ring the changes by using shredded spring greens instead of pak choi.

Makes 4 portions

2 tbsp sunflower oil
1 bunch of spring onions, trimmed and
    cut in short lengths
2 celery sticks, cut in matchsticks
450g skinless chicken breast or thigh
    meat, cut in short strips

1 garlic clove, crushed
½ tsp five-spice powder
2.5cm piece fresh root ginger, grated
175g shiitake mushrooms, sliced
4 heads pak choi (about 400g),
    coarsely shredded
4 tbsp soy sauce

1. Heat the oil in a wok or a large frying pan. Add the spring onions and celery and stir-fry for 1 minute. Add the chicken and stir-fry for 2 minutes.
2. Add the garlic, five-spice powder, ginger, and mushrooms and stir-fry all the ingredients together for 1 minute.
3. Add the pak choi and stir-fry for a further minute. Add the soy sauce, toss for 30 seconds, and serve.

Lunch only
Add 4 nests (200g) wholewheat Chinese noodles (reduce the quantity of chicken to 350g and the mushrooms to 115g for the stir-fry). Cook according to the packet directions while you make the stir-fry. Drain the noodles, pile them into bowls, and spoon the stir-fry on top.

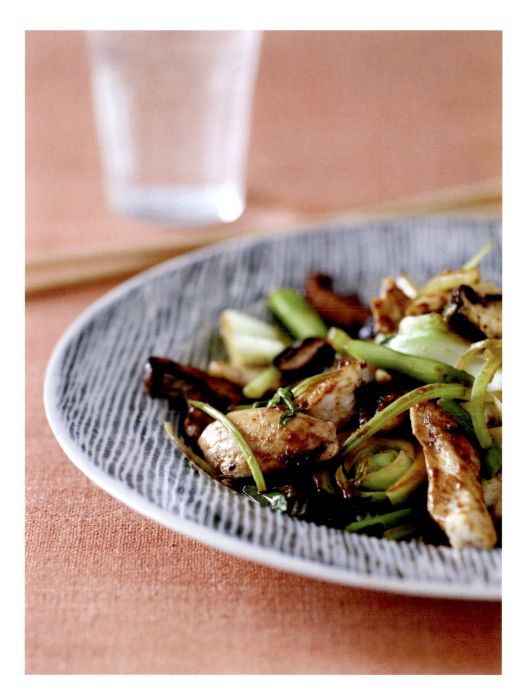

Duck, goose, and feathered game

The meat of all these birds (which also includes grouse, pheasant, partridge, pigeon, guinea fowl, and quail) is darker in appearance than chicken, and richer in flavour. Careful cooking is needed to ensure they remain tender and succulent. Being more expensive than chicken and turkey, they may not be everyday dishes, but they make delicious eating. Duck, quail, guinea fowl, and pigeon are available all year, goose is mostly reared for Christmas, and wild game birds are sold only in season. Duck and goose flesh should be firm and moist, but not wet, when you buy it.

Ducks and geese have a large layer of fat beneath their skin, which should be drained off once the meat is cooked. And although the crispy skin may taste delicious, it, like chicken and turkey skin, is high in calories and should be removed before eating. Since they contain so much fat, duck and geese with their skin on need nothing added to keep them succulent as they cook.

Three simple cooking techniques

Grill Only suitable for breasts or spatchcocked birds (split in half through the backbone and opened out flat). Remove the skin. Brush with oil or marinate first, if you like, then put some foil in the base of a grill pan to collect the juices. Grill for 2–8 minutes per side (depending on size) until golden brown but still pink in the centre (do not overcook).

Sauté Suitable for breasts or spatchcocked birds (see above) only. Remove the skin. Heat 1–2 tablespoons of oil in a frying pan. Sauté for 2–8 minutes per side (depending on size) until golden brown but pink in the centre. Do not overcook the meat.

Casserole Brown small whole birds or diced game meat quickly in a little oil with a chopped onion in a flameproof casserole or large saucepan. Add vegetables of your choice. Cover with half chicken stock, half apple juice, season, and add some herbs or other flavourings. Bring to the boil, cover, then either reduce the heat and simmer very gently, or transfer to the oven at 160°C (Gas 3) for 40 minutes–1 hour or until tender.

Meal suggestions

- Grilled marinated duck breasts (marinate the breasts first in olive oil, balsamic vinegar, some chopped onion, and fresh sage) with fresh watercress and mashed swede (for lunch, add sautéed potatoes)
- Roast duck or goose (stuffed with a few sage leaves) with roasted onions, carrots, and broccoli, and gravy made from the giblet stock and pan juices with all the fat poured off (for lunch, add new potatoes)
- Roast pheasant or duck with roasted fennel or celery, Jerusalem artichoke purée and gravy made with the pan juices, stock, and a dash of balsamic vinegar (for lunch, add roasted potatoes)
- Roast grouse or pheasant with chestnuts and braised red cabbage with beetroot (for lunch, add sweet potato mash)
- Duck, pigeon, or pheasant breast strips, stir-fried with sliced spring onions and garlic. Add cherry tomatoes and bean sprouts at the last minute and moisten with soy sauce and a splash of rice vinegar. Serve on a bed of steamed pak choi (for lunch, add Chinese wholewheat noodles).
- Partridge, quail, or pigeon casserole with turnips and mushrooms, cooked in equal amounts of chicken stock and apple juice, and served on a bed of shredded steamed spring greens (for lunch, add jacket potatoes)

Snack suggestions

- Diced cold duck, goose, or game meat mixed with grated raw or chopped cooked beetroot, moistened with balsamic vinegar, in half a pitta bread
- Shredded cold duck meat spread over 1/2 or 1 corn tortilla with julienne strips of carrot, cucumber, and spring onion, with a dash of soy sauce and white balsamic, and rolled into a Chinese-style pancake
- Diced cold duck, goose, or game meat with a couple of spoonfuls of cooked sweetcorn, moistened with a little mayonnaise and flavoured with a dash of curry paste, spooned into a halved, deseeded red pepper
- A cold duck or game leg (or 2 if very small), skin removed, with some cornichons and cherry tomatoes

What to look for
- Duck: sold fresh or frozen as breast fillets or legs, or whole
- Pheasants and pigeon: breast fillets or whole
- Other game birds: whole to roast or braise

Ways to cook or serve
- Grill
- Roast
- Sauté
- Casserole

Simple ways to flavour
- Herbs (chopped fresh): sage mixed with onion for duck and goose dishes
- Spices: nutmeg, cinnamon, mace, star anise, and Chinese five-spice, or a cajun spice rub (sweet and smoked paprika, cayenne, black pepper, garlic, dried oregano, and thyme mixed together)
- Beetroot, Jerusalem artichoke, and turnips, all roasted or puréed, and minted peas or mangetout

Warm duck breast salad with beetroot and mangetout

This salad is equally good made with pigeon, pheasant, or partridge breasts when they are in season and available to buy.

Makes 4 portions

115g mangetout, trimmed
4 skinless duck breasts
Freshly ground black pepper
4 tbsp olive oil
1 x 410g can cannellini beans in water
   (or 240g cooked [115g raw weight]
   beans), drained and heated

A handful of halved cherry tomatoes
1 x 70g packet lamb's lettuce
4 spring onions, chopped
½ cucumber, peeled and diced
2 raw beetroot, peeled and shredded
2 tbsp balsamic vinegar
4 tbsp pure apple juice
2 tsp fresh thyme leaves

1. Spread the mangetout out evenly in a metal colander or steamer, cover, and steam for just 1½ minutes to soften. Then set aside.
2. Season the duck breasts well with black pepper. Heat the oil in a frying pan and fry the breasts quickly for 2 minutes on each side to brown them. Then turn down the heat, cover the pan, and cook for a further minute until just firm but still slightly pink in the centre. Remove the duck from the pan, wrap it in kitchen foil, and leave it to one side to rest.
3. Mix the cannellini beans, tomatoes, lamb's lettuce, spring onions, cucumber, and mangetout together and pile on plates. Scatter the beetroot over the top. Carve the duck into slices and arrange on top of the salad.
4. Quickly add the vinegar, apple juice and half the thyme to the juices in the pan. Bring to the boil, stir, and season to taste. Spoon over the salad, sprinkle with the remaining thyme, and serve straight away.

Lunch only
Add 450g baby new potatoes, scrubbed.
Boil the potatoes in water with just a pinch of salt added, if you like, for about 12 minutes until tender. When cooked, drain, return to the pan, and put the lid on. Set aside while you cook the duck. Then mix the potatoes with the lamb's lettuce, spring onions, cucumber, and mangetout.

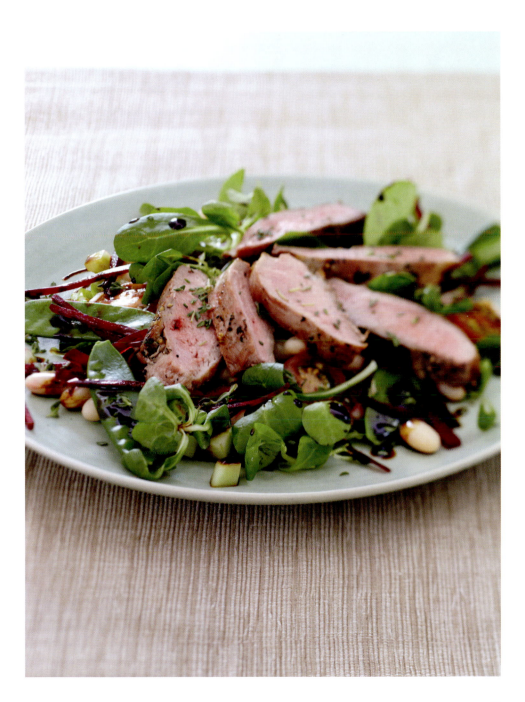

Eggs

Arguably the ultimate fast food, eggs are are extremely quick and easy to cook if you want an instant meal. They can be used as an ingredient in other dishes (such as beaten with a little milk or half-fat crème fraîche and added to pasta after cooking and draining to make a creamy sauce). Many people have a concern about eating eggs due to their dietary cholesterol content, but as long as the rest of your diet is low in saturated fats and simple carbohydrates, the cholesterol in eggs should have little impact on overall cholesterol levels in the blood. There may be some subtle nutritional differences between the various types of eggs on offer, but for our purposes whatever type of egg you choose is suitable.

Duck eggs have more protein in their whites than hens eggs and tend to go tough when boiled, so are best coddled instead (below). They also make great soufflés. Avoid buying tubs of egg mayonnaise, as the fat content is unnecessarily high, and most recipes contain sugar (bought mayonnaise is fine if it is sugar-free).

Three simple cooking techniques

Coddle/boil To coddle, put the egg or eggs in a pan, cover with cold water, bring to the boil, cover with a lid, remove from the heat, and leave to stand (8 minutes for hens eggs, 12 minutes for ducks). To boil, put an egg in a small pan, cover with cold water, bring to the boil, cover with a lid, and boil for:
Hens eggs – 31/2 minutes for soft-boiled, 5–7 minutes for hard-boiled
Quails eggs – 1 minute only for soft-boiled, 3 minutes for hard
Goose eggs – 11 minutes for hard-boiled (too big to serve soft-boiled).

Poach Use very fresh eggs. Bring a frying pan of water to the boil, add 1 table-spoon of vinegar or lemon juice, turn down to a gentle simmer, break an egg into a cup, then slide it out of the cup into the water. Fold the white over the yolk with a spoon. Cover and cook for 2 minutes or until the white is firm and the yolk still soft. Cook longer for firmer eggs. Lift out with a slotted spoon.

Omelette Put 2–3 eggs in a bowl, season, add a splash of water, fresh herbs if you like, and whisk. Heat a knob of butter in a frying pan and, when foaming, add the eggs. Cook, lifting and stirring, until partially set. Add flavourings of your choice. When the base is golden brown and the top is creamy and almost set, tilt the pan, fold the omelette over, and slide it onto a plate.

Meal suggestions

▸ Salade Niçoise: quartered hard-boiled eggs on a salad of lettuce, capers, anchovies, tomatoes, cucumber, and sliced red onion, dressed with a little French dressing (for lunch, add diced cooked new potatoes)

▸ Omelette filled with a little grated cheese, chopped ham, and sliced cooked mushrooms, and served with a mixed salad (for lunch, add a slice of wholegrain bread or toast)

▸ Quick eggs florentine: poach the eggs, arrange on a bed of wilted spinach and sliced tomatoes in a flameproof dish, sprinkle with grated cheese, and brown briefly under a preheated grill (for lunch, add wholemeal muffins).

▸ Scrambled eggs and smoked salmon with a large mixed salad (for lunch, add wholegrain toast)

▸ Quick Cuban eggs: sauté sliced peppers, onions, and tomatoes in a little olive oil in a pan until soft. Season and flavour with dried oregano and a pinch of chilli powder. Serve topped with fried eggs (for lunch, serve with rolled up wholewheat tortillas).

Snack suggestions

▸ 1 slice of cold omelette with diced vegetables and a slice of wholegrain bread

▸ 1 small slice of cold frittata (pp. 44–45), or bought frittata, with a sliced tomato

▸ 1 chopped hard-boiled egg mixed with a little mayonnaise and some salad cress on 2 oatcakes

▸ A soft-boiled egg with baby corn cob 'soldiers'

What to look for
•Barn-laid hens eggs
•Omega 3 hens eggs
•Organic and free-range hens, quails, duck, goose, and ostrich eggs (1 ostrich egg is equivalent to 18–24 hens eggs)

Ways to cook or serve
•Boil
•Scramble
•Poach
•Omelette
•Coddle
•Fry

Simple ways to flavour
•Mediterranean flavours: tomatoes, peppers, anchovies, olives, garlic, onions, lemon
•Herbs: fresh parsley, tarragon, or dill, dried oregano
•Spices: curry powder
•Cheeses, ham, lean back bacon, leeks, spinach, smoked fish, mushrooms, tomatoes, prawns

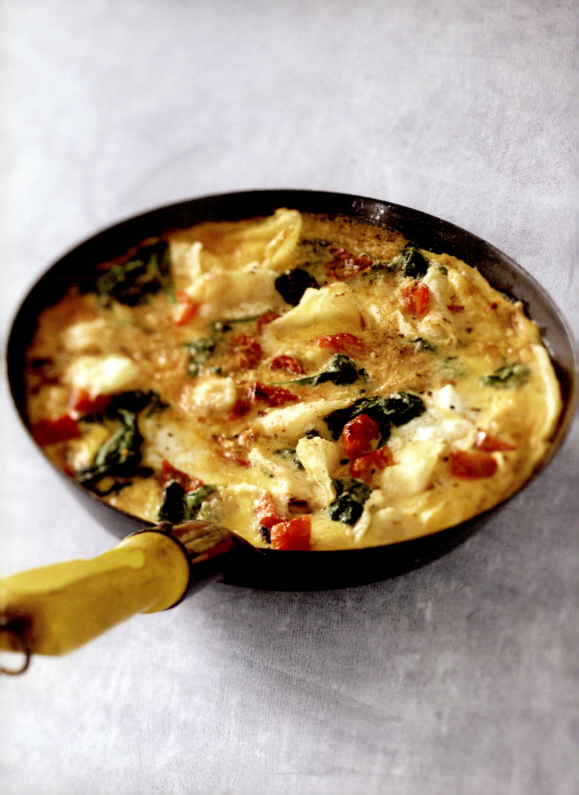

Spinach and cottage cheese frittata

This omelette cake is great as a warm dish for supper, but it is also good cold in a packed lunch. If you want to eat a side dish with it, try a tomato and onion salad.

Makes 4 portions

2 tbsp olive oil
1 celeriac, peeled, quartered, and
 thinly sliced
115g baby leaf spinach
115g low-fat plain cottage cheese
55g sun-ripened tomatoes, cut into
 small pieces

2 tbsp freshly grated Parmesan or
 other hard Italian cheese
Freshly grated nutmeg
Freshly ground black pepper
6 eggs, beaten

To serve: tomato and onion salad

1. Heat the oil in a large non-stick frying pan. Add the celeriac and cook over a low heat, stirring and turning gently until it is coated in oil and softening. Cover with a lid or foil and cook as gently as possible until the celeriac is really soft and breaking up, but not brown – about 20 minutes – stirring and turning occasionally.
2. Meanwhile, wash the spinach well and shake off the excess water. Cook in a separate pan without any added water, tossing lightly until wilted, about 3 minutes. Drain thoroughly in a colander and squeeze out all excess moisture. Chop with scissors.
3. When the celeriac is soft, scatter over the spinach, cottage cheese, and sun-ripened tomatoes. Sprinkle over the grated cheese and dust with freshly grated nutmeg and lots of freshly ground black pepper. Mix well, then stir in the beaten eggs and cook, lifting and stirring until the frittata is beginning to set. Cover the pan and cook gently until the eggs are almost set and the base is golden (about 5 minutes).
4. Meanwhile, preheat the grill. When the eggs are nearly set, put the pan under the grill to brown the top, about 5 minutes. Remove from the grill. Leave to cool for at least 5 minutes. Serve warm or cold, cut in wedges.

Lunch only
Substitute 3 fairly large, scrubbed potatoes for the celeriac.

Beef

Red meat isn't always associated with good health, but it is a good source of protein as well as other essential nutrients. As long as the beef you buy is lean, there is no reason to exclude it from your diet: just over a quarter of the calories of a lean cut of beef are 'fat calories' (p.17), and less than half of those comprise saturated fat.

Beef is succulent and tasty so it is delicious plainly cooked, but it will also take on robust flavours such as horseradish or chilli. With the exception of cheaper stewing cuts, most dishes and cuts of beef can be cooked simply and quickly with tasty, filling results. The creamy fat that surrounds red meat is a significant source of saturated fats, so trim away as much of it as you can before you cook it and cut off the rest before eating. Beef should be dark, not bright, red. Avoid if dry or grey at the edges or if it has thick bands of gristle, cheap mince (it will be full of fat and will not taste good), and processed bought products such as sausages and burgers.

Three simple cooking techniques

Grill Brush with oil, season with freshly ground black pepper, and grill for 2–3 minutes each side for rare, 3–4 minutes each side for medium, 6–8 minutes each side for well done (depending on thickness). The touch test is: if wobbly, it is very rare; if slightly spongy, it is medium-cooked; if firm, it is well done.

Pot Roast Brown a joint of beef in a little sunflower oil on all sides in a flame-proof casserole. Remove from the dish. Add diced onions and root vegetables and soften slightly, stirring. Top with the meat, season, add other flavourings such as a bouquet garni, pour in some beef stock, bring to the boil, cover, and cook in the oven at 160°C (Gas 3) for about 4 hours until tender.

Carpaccio Roll a piece of beef fillet in crushed peppercorns. Wrap tightly in clingfilm and freeze for 2 hours only. Unwrap and cut into wafer-thin slices with a sharp knife. Store in the fridge and eat within 24 hours, or layer the slices with baking parchment or cling film, wrap, and freeze. To eat, arrange the slices on a plate with a pile of rocket in the centre. Sprinkle with Parmesan or other Italian hard cheese shavings, a drizzle of olive oil and lemon juice, and serve with cherry or baby plum tomatoes. (For lunch, add brown bread.)

Meal suggestions

▶ Roast beef with carrots, leafy greens, and gravy made from the well-drained meat juices and beef stock (for lunch, add roast or new potatoes)

▶ Grilled steak (marinated first, if you like; see Simple ways to flavour, right) with a mixed salad (for lunch, add potato wedges, p.144, or a jacket potato)

▶ Beef and vegetable stir-fry with mushrooms and bean sprouts (for lunch, add soba [buckwheat] or udon [brown rice] noodles)

▶ Beef stew with root vegetables and broad beans (for lunch, add potatoes to the stew)

▶ Sizzling steak or liver salad with avocado: stir-fry strips of tender beef or calves liver for 2–3 minutes in a little olive oil, toss in some balsamic vinegar and chopped fresh herbs, season, and pile onto a large mixed salad with sliced avocado (for lunch add cold, cooked wholemeal penne pasta, Camargue red rice, or brown rice).

Snack suggestions

▶ 1 slice of cold roast beef on a piece of wholemeal bread spread with a scraping of mustard and mayonnaise (instead of butter) and topped with lettuce and/or sliced tomato

▶ 4 wafer-thin slices of cooked beef on 2 oatcakes topped with a dot of horseradish and some chopped cornichons

▶ 1 wholemeal chappati or flatbread spread thinly with tapenade (chopped olive paste), with a thin slice of beef and grated carrot on top, and rolled into a wrap

▶ 2–4 slices of beef carpaccio (see left, or buy vacuum-packed) on a large wholegrain cracker, spread with a scraping of low-fat soft white cheese and a squeeze of lemon juice

What to look for
•Roasting: topside, top rump, sirloin, or rib
•Grilling: rump, sirloin, fillet, rib-eye, veal chops, or escalopes
•Stir-frying: fillet, rump, sirloin, frying steak, or calves liver
•Pot-roasting: brisket or silverside
•Stews or casseroles: braising or stewing steak (e.g. shin, chuck, blade, skirt, or flank, and also kidney or heart)
•Lean minced beef

Ways to cook or serve
•Roast
•Grill
•Stir-fry
•Pot roast
•Stew, casserole, or curry
•Carpaccio
•Burgers and meatballs

Simple ways to flavour
•Condiments: horseradish, various mustards
•Marinade: olive oil, red-wine vinegar, a splash of apple juice, garlic, and chopped herbs
•Mushrooms, onions, carrots, tomatoes, olives, peppers

Braised steak with olives and tomatoes

Serve with leafy green vegetables, such as shredded greens, steamed or boiled in just a small amount of water for a few minutes just before the casserole is ready.

Makes 4 portions

2 tbsp olive oil
675g piece of lean braising steak, trimmed of all fat and cut in 4 equal pieces or bite-sized chunks
2 onions, chopped
1 garlic clove, crushed
1 small butternut squash, cut in bite-sized chunks
1 large carrot, cut in chunky slices
2 beefsteak tomatoes, skinned and chopped

4 canned anchovy fillets, finely chopped, or 2 tsp anchovy essence or paste
16 stoned black olives, drained
450ml beef stock
150ml tomato juice
2 tbsp tomato purée
Finely grated zest of 1 small orange
1 tsp dried oregano
1 bay leaf
Freshly ground black pepper
A little chopped parsley, to garnish

To serve: steamed or boiled leafy green vegetables

1. Preheat the oven to 160°C (Gas 3). Heat the oil in a large flameproof casserole. Add the beef and fry on all sides to brown. Remove from the pan with a slotted spoon and reserve.
2. Add the onions, garlic, squash, and carrots to the pan and fry quickly for 2 minutes, stirring all the while. Return the beef to the casserole and add the tomatoes, anchovy fillets, essence, or paste, and olives.
3. Blend the stock with the tomato juice, tomato purée, and orange zest and pour over the meat. Add the oregano and bay leaf and season well with freshly ground black pepper.
4. Bring to the boil, cover, and cook in the oven for 2 hours until the meat is meltingly tender and the sauce is rich and thick. Taste and re-season, if necessary. Garnish with chopped parsley and serve.

Lunch only
Serve with baked jacket potatoes.

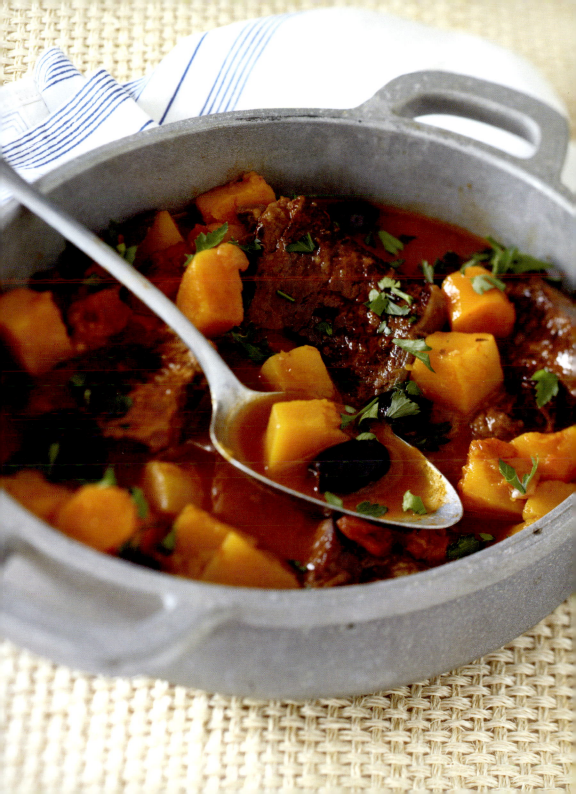

Lamb, goat, and venison
Although venison is technically game, rather than a red meat like lamb and goat, it is now farmed in this country and can be cooked in similar ways. Lambs or kids are animals under a year old; between one and two years old, lamb is called hogget and goat chevron. If over two years old, lamb – and sometimes goat – is called mutton.

Lamb can be a fatty meat, so trim the meat well before cooking it. Goat and venison, on the other hand, are very lean (before roasting, for example, they should be well-rubbed with oil so they don't dry out, and venison steaks shouldn't be overcooked or they become really tough). Browning meat quickly, then wrapping it in foil and finishing it off briefly in the oven (pan-roasting) produces meltingly tender results with venison, and works wonderfully with lamb and goat, too (see below). When choosing a cut of meat, all three types should look and smell fresh. The flesh should be moist, not wet, and any fat should feel firm, not slimy.

Three simple cooking techniques

Pan-roast Heat a little sunflower or olive oil in a frying pan. Season steaks with freshly ground black pepper (marinate first, if you like; see Simple ways to flavour, opposite). Brown for 1–2 minutes a side (depending on thickness), then wrap in foil and roast in the oven at 150°C (Gas 2) for 10 minutes. Remove and leave to stand for 5 minutes, then serve with the juices from the foil. If marinated, pour the marinade into the pan, boil briefly, and spoon over.

Curry Brown onions, garlic, and diced lamb, goat, or venison in a little olive or sunflower oil in a large saucepan. Stir in curry paste to taste. Add a bay leaf, some mushrooms if you like, enough lamb or beef stock to cover, and half a block of creamed coconut. Bring to the boil, stirring, reduce the heat, and cover and simmer gently until thick and tender. Season to taste. Add some fresh spinach at the last minute if you like, and stir until wilted.

Burgers Mix minced lamb, goat, or venison (allow 100g per burger) with finely chopped onion, fresh thyme, seasoning, and beaten egg to bind. Shape into burgers, brush with a little oil and grill on foil on a grill rack, or heat a tablespoon of oil in a non-stick frying pan and fry, pressing them down with a fish slice. Allow 6 minutes on each side, or until cooked through and golden.

Meal suggestions

▸ Roast lamb, goat, or venison with mixed roasted vegetables, cabbage, and gravy made from the well-drained meat juices, lamb stock, and a splash of soy sauce (for lunch, add roast or new potatoes)

▸ Grilled chops (marinated first, if you like; see Simple ways to flavour, right) with condiments (see Simple ways to flavour) and a mixed salad (for lunch, add some fluffy mashed potato)

▸ Pan-roasted steaks with mushrooms and cherry tomatoes (cooked in the foil with the meat) with green beans (for lunch, add some new potatoes)

▸ Lamb, goat, or venison curry with cucumber and radish sambal (p.189) without the peanuts (for lunch, add brown basmati rice)

▸ Lamb, goat, or venison stew with leeks, carrots, and turnips. Add star anise and fresh chopped chilli, if you like, for an Asian flavour (for lunch, add large chunks of potato or sweet potato to the stew when cooking)

Snack suggestions

▸ A spoonful of chopped cooked lamb, goat, or venison mixed with a little natural unsweetened yoghurt and mint and a few spices of cucumber in half a wholewheat pitta bread

▸ A cold slice of lambs or goats liver, chopped, mixed with some soft cheese and herbs, spread on wholewheat crackers

▸ Some diced cooked lamb, goat, or venison mixed with a little mayonnaise and curry paste, spread on a wholemeal chapatti or flatbread topped with some lettuce and rolled up

What to look for
•Roasting: leg, shoulder, rack, chops (lamb and goat), haunch and saddle (venison)
•Grilling: chops, steaks, liver, kidneys
•Stir-frying and sautéing: fillet, leg steaks, lamb or goat kidneys and liver
•Stews, casseroles, or curries: diced braising meat, usually from the shoulder or leg (also sold as mince), neck chops (lamb and goat), lamb or goat shanks

Ways to cook or serve
•Roast
•Grill
•Stir-fry or sauté
•Pan-roast
•Stew, casserole or curry
•Burgers/meatballs

Simple ways to flavour
•Condiments: for lamb, make a mint sauce with plenty of chopped fresh mint, a splash of apple juice, and balsamic vinegar. For goat and venison, try a chestnut purée flavoured with nutmeg or cinnamon
•Spices: chilli, fenugreek, cardamom, cumin, coriander, cinnamon, Thai or Indian curry pastes, harissa or sambal oelek
•Herbs: fresh thyme, oregano, mint, rosemary, coriander, bay
•Marinade: olive oil, balsamic vinegar, chopped onion and/or garlic, chopped rosemary or thyme, a piece of cinnamon stick and a bay leaf

Pan-roasted venison steak with rosemary and garlic

Venison steaks are best quickly seared and then allowed to finish cooking briefly in a low oven to tenderise the meat. This is equally good made with lamb leg steaks or neck fillet.

Makes 4 portions

4 venison steaks
1 tbsp olive oil
Freshly ground black pepper
1 tsp juniper berries, crushed
2 garlic cloves, finely chopped
1 tbsp balsamic vinegar
150ml beef stock

To serve: baby carrots

1 tbsp soy sauce
A few fresh rosemary leaves
  to garnish (optional)

For the pea purée:
350g shelled young fresh or
  frozen peas
4 tbsp half-fat crème fraîche

1. Wipe the meat with kitchen towel and rub it all over with the oil. Place it in a container with a lid and season well with black pepper. Sprinkle all over with the juniper, and garlic. Cover and leave at room temperature to marinate for 1 hour.
2. Preheat the oven to 150°C (Gas 2). Heat a griddle pan or non-stick frying pan. Fry the steaks quickly for 1 minute on each side to brown (if you don't like your meat too rare, cook for 2 minutes each side, but no more). Wrap the meat in foil and place the parcel on an ovenproof plate or baking sheet. Cook in the oven for 10 minutes, then remove immediately. Set the pan aside to make the sauce later.
3. Meanwhile, heat 150ml of water to just cover the base of a saucepan. Add the peas as the water boils, cover, and cook for 4–5 minutes, stirring occasionally until the peas are tender. Then remove the lid and boil rapidly to evaporate any remaining water. Remove the pan from the heat and in a blender, or using a hand blender in the pan, purée the peas with the crème fraîche. Season with black pepper.
4. Add the balsamic vinegar, beef stock, and soy sauce to the pan that the venison was browned in and boil for 2 minutes until reduced by half, scraping up any sediment. Add any juices from the foil parcel. Slice the steaks or leave whole.
5. Spoon the purée onto warm plates. Top each with a venison steak and a sprig of rosemary, if using. Spoon the pan juices over and serve with the baby carrots.

Lunch only
Serve with new potatoes.

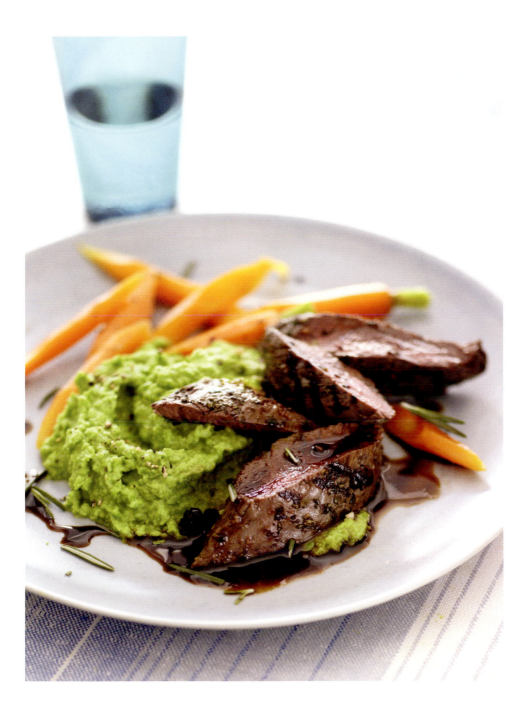

Pork and veal
Although these meats are from different animals – pigs and male dairy calves – they can be cooked in similar ways. Pork should be well-trimmed of fat before you eat it, and pork crackling is very high in saturated fat, so you should avoid it. Veal is much lower in fat than pork. Both meats should have a good pink colour when you buy them, the pork fat should be white, and any rind should be dry. Belly pork can be very fatty, but is inexpensive. Only buy if it is lean.

Raw cured ham is usually served very thin and is excellent cooked as well as raw. Cooked ham and some cured bacon can have lots of additives and sugar, so check before you buy. Always choose lean slices (avoid streaky bacon and pancetta as they has too much fat) and trim off fat before use. Don't eat these products too often, as they contain a lot of added salt.

Three simple cooking techniques

Sauté Dip thin slices of meat in beaten egg, then in ground almonds mixed with a pinch of dried herbs and seasoning (for lunch, use breadcrumbs instead of almonds). Fry in a couple of tablespoons of olive or sunflower oil over a moderate heat until golden and cooked through (2–3 minutes a side).

Griddle Brush the meat with a little oil and season lightly. Preheat the griddle pan until it is very hot when you hold your hand 5cm above the pan. Lay the chops or steaks in the pan and fry for 6 minutes, turn over, and cook the other side until the meat is cooked through and striped brown. Don't prod the meat with a fork or knife to check for doneness or the juices will run out and the meat will be tough. When cooked, it should feel firm to the touch, but not hard. Deglaze the pan with a little stock, if you like.

Paté Mix minced pork or veal and minced pigs liver (you need about 500g in all) with minced onion, garlic, and chopped fresh sage. Stir in some crème fraîche. Season well. Mix with beaten egg. Pack into a greased loaf tin and cover with greaseproof paper and then foil, twisting and folding under the rim of the tin to secure. Bake in a roasting tin with enough water to come halfway up the sides of the loaf tin for 1 1/2 hours at 160°C (Gas 3) until firm to the touch. Remove from the oven and weigh down the top with cans of food or scale weights. Leave until cold, then chill before turning out and slicing.

Meal suggestions

- Roast pork or veal with root vegetable mash, broccoli, and gravy made from the meat juices (spoon the fat off first) and beef stock (for lunch, add roast or new potatoes)
- Griddled steak or chop (marinate first– see below right – if you like, then dry well with kitchen paper) with a mixed salad (for lunch, add some new potatoes)
- Pork and cashew stir-fry with ready-prepared stir-fry vegetables flavoured with garlic, Chinese five-spice, and soy sauce (for lunch, add wholewheat noodles)
- Pork or veal and butter bean stew with onions, carrots, swede, and canned chopped tomatoes and flavoured with cinnamon and garlic (for lunch, spoon over brown or red rice)
- Pork or veal escalopes. Sauté (see opposite) and serve with warmed passata flavoured with fresh chopped basil and green beans or broccoli (for lunch, add some wholewheat noodles).

Snack suggestions

- 1 slice of lean cold roast pork or veal on half a wholemeal bagel, spread with some mayonnaise, flavoured with a little grainy mustard, and topped with sliced cucumber
- A little diced chopped pork or veal with some chopped beetroot in a little natural yoghurt in half a wholemeal pitta bread
- A small slice of pork or veal pâté (see opposite) on a slice of wholegrain toast with a scraping of English mustard and some cherry tomatoes

What to look for
- Roasting: leg, loin, shoulder, spare rib joint, trimmed spare ribs (pork), belly (pork, lean)
- Stir-frying and sautéing: fillet (tenderloin), chops, escalopes (thin slices from the leg), liver, kidneys
- Grilling: chops, leg steaks, escalopes, fillet (tenderloin)
- Stewing and casseroling: pork hock, diced braising meat, usually from the shoulder, belly, liver, kidneys
- Lean minced pork, veal

Ways to cook
- Roast
- Stir-fry or sauté
- Grill
- Griddle
- Stew, casserole, or curry
- Burgers and meatballs
- Pâté made from minced meat and liver (pigs liver only; calves liver is expensive and is better stir-fried, sautéed, or grilled)

Simple ways to flavour
- Herbs: fresh sage with onions is excellent for stuffing and in stir-fries, pâtés, and stews
- Spices: paprika, cinnamon, cloves, and star anise in stews and casseroles
- Marinade: olive oil, white balsamic, garlic, coriander seeds, and leaves
- Dried beans, lentils and chick-peas with pork

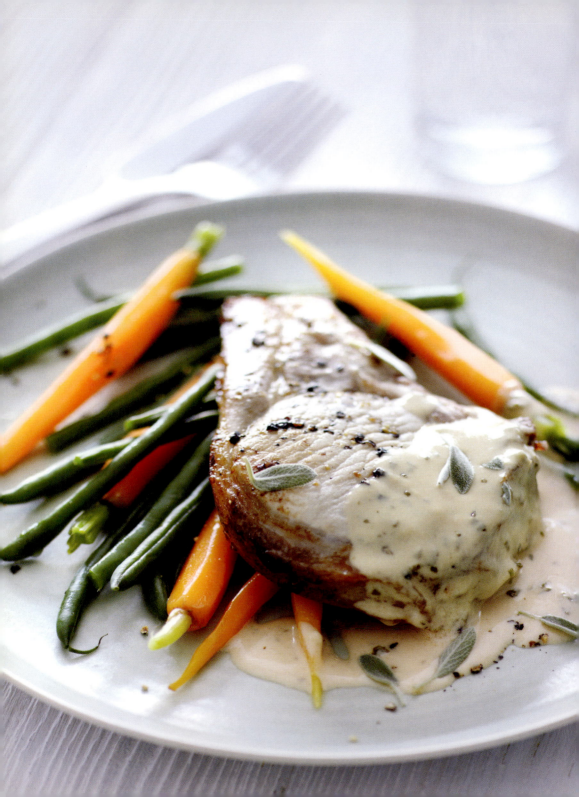

Grilled pork chops with sage and mustard sauce

Don't be tempted to keep pricking these pork chops or they become stringy and tough. Trim them of excess fat before cooking. To turn this into a more substantial evening meal, make some mashed celeriac to go with it.

Makes 4 portions

4 pork chops on the bone, trimmed
1 tbsp olive oil
Freshly ground black pepper
120ml pure apple juice

2 tbsp chopped fresh sage
200ml half-fat crème fraîche
1 tbsp Dijon mustard
4 small fresh sage sprigs to garnish

To serve: carrots and green beans

1. Line the grill pan with foil and preheat the grill. Brush the pork chops with the oil and season with lots of black pepper. Grill the chops for 8–10 minutes on each side until golden and cooked through. Then wrap the chops in foil and keep the parcel warm while you make the sauce.
2. Carefully lift out the foil from the grill pan and tip any juices into a small pan, scraping any sediment from the foil into the pan, too. Add the apple juice and sage and boil rapidly until reduced by half: about 1 minute. Stir in the crème fraîche and mustard and heat, stirring, until bubbling. Taste and re-season, if necessary.
3. Place a pork chop on each plate and spoon the sauce over. Garnish with tiny sprigs of fresh sage and serve with the carrots and green beans.

Lunch only
Make mashed potato flavoured with fresh snipped chives.

Cheese

There are countless varieties of cheeses now available, but the main question to ask in the context of this eating plan is whether you should include full-fat cheese in your snacks and meals or stick to low-fat options. The rule of thumb here is that smaller amounts of full-fat cheese, such as Cheddar, can be used as a snack when eaten with a complex carbohydrate, such as bread, but when larger amounts of cheese are called for, such as including cheese in a large salad for a main meal, low-fat or a reduced-fat cheese is the better choice.

It's also important to vary your choices and not eat full-fat cheese every day.

Goats cheese, Edam, and mozzarella are all lower in fat than most cheeses, and are a better choice that many low-fat versions of familar cheeses that are now available in supermarkets.

Three simple cooking techniques

Grill For cheese on toast, cover a slice of toast with a small handful of grated melting cheese such as Cheddar, and place under the grill. Grill for 3–5 minutes or until melted, bubbling, and turning golden. To grill thick slices of halloumi, goats cheese, or bloomed white cheese such as Camembert wedges, brush with olive oil, place on oiled foil on the grill rack, and grill until just melting and turning golden on top – about 2–3 minutes. Do not turn over. Serve immediately.

Bake Cover cooked vegetables with grated cheese in an ovenproof dish. Sprinkle with a few chopped nuts (or, if for lunch, top with crushed cornflakes). Bake at 190°C (Gas 5) until the cheese melts and bubbles: about 30 minutes.

Sauce A cheese sauce to serve at lunchtime with macaroni, fish, or vegetables: put 3 tablespoons of plain flour in a small saucepan. Blend in 250ml of milk with a wire whisk until smooth. Add a knob of butter and a bay leaf. Bring to the boil, whisking all the time, and cook for 2 minutes, still whisking until thick and smooth. Discard the bay leaf. Stir in 2 handfuls of strong grated Cheddar cheese or other melting cheese. Season to taste. For evening meals, use the quick crème fraîche cheese sauce on page 165.

Meal suggestions

▸ Tricolour salad: sliced mozzarella, sliced tomatoes, avocado, and a handful of rocket drizzled with olive oil and lemon juice and a good grinding of black pepper (for lunch, add wholegrain bread)

▸ Greek village salad with feta cheese: shredded white cabbage and lettuce, diced tomatoes, cucumber, sliced onion separated into rings, black olives, crumbled feta cheese, and a dusting of dried oregano, drizzed with olive oil and red-wine vinegar (for lunch, add wholemeal pitta breads)

▸ Grilled goats cheese on a bed of quickly sautéed shredded leeks with diced cooked beetroot, with a handful of walnuts and baby leaf spinach thrown in at the last minute and tossed in a little French dressing (for lunch, add couscous)

▸ Cheese soup: cook diced carrots, celeriac or swede, and onion in vegetable stock with some chopped thyme. Purée the vegetables, return them to the pan, add a little strong Cheddar, some milk, and chopped parsley, season, and reheat (for lunch, add wholegrain bagels).

▸ Courgette and ham gratin: steam or boil sliced courgettes, put in a flameproof dish with some diced ham and some halved cherry tomatoes. Sprinkle with some chopped sage and seasoning. Top with cottage cheese and little grated Parmesan or other hard Italian cheese and bake or grill until golden.

Snack suggestions

▸ Grated Edam and carrot with a chopped pickled onion in half a wholemeal pitta bread

▸ Soft goats cheese spread on thin slices of cooked beetroot on 2 oatcakes

▸ Cottage cheese mixed with chopped red pepper, diced cucumber, chopped celery, and freshly ground black pepper

▸ A finger of hard cheese, such as Cheddar, with an apple or pear

Protein

What to look for
• Lower in fat: goats cheese, Edam, and mozzarella
• Low-fat cheeses: feta, halloumi, cottage cheese
• Cheese for cooked dishes: Parmesan, pecorino, and Grana Padano (all Italian hard cheeses), blue cheeses (as they have fairly strong flavours, so smaller quantities are needed; this is also true if you use a strong mature Cheddar rather than a mild one)

Ways to cook or serve
• Grill
• Bake
• Grate
• Sauce
• Salad

Simple ways to flavour
• Walnuts, hazelnuts, and peanuts all enhance cheese and give added crunch
• Celery, tomatoes, beetroot, fresh and pickled onions

Toasted halloumi and pine nut salad

Halloumi is a wonderful firm, almost meaty, cheese that browns and softens when grilled, but doesn't melt. Serve the salad as soon as the cheese is toasted, as it hardens again as it cools.

Makes 4 portions

2 tbsp pine nuts
2 baby red onions
250g block halloumi cheese,
    cut into 8 slices
3 tbsp olive oil
1 x 70g packet wild rocket

12 baby plum tomatoes, halved
8 baby corn cobs, cut in short lengths
2 tsp lemon juice
2 tbsp chopped fresh tarragon
2 tbsp chopped fresh parsley
Freshly ground black pepper

1. Preheat the grill. Heat a small frying pan and toast the pine nuts briefly, tossing them in the pan until lightly golden. Then tip them onto a plate and set aside.
2. Slice the unpeeled red onions and separate into rings, discarding the skin and outer layer. Place in a large bowl.
3. Cut the halloumi slices in halves lengthways. Place on foil on the grill rack and brush with a little of the olive oil.
4. Put the rocket, tomatoes, and corn in with the onions. Add the remaining olive oil and the lemon juice, tarragon, parsley, and a good grinding of black pepper. Toss gently and pile on four plates.
5. Quickly toast the halloumi, close to the heat source, on one side only until lightly golden – about 3 minutes. Transfer to the salads and scatter the pine nuts over the top.

Lunch only
Serve with wholemeal bread

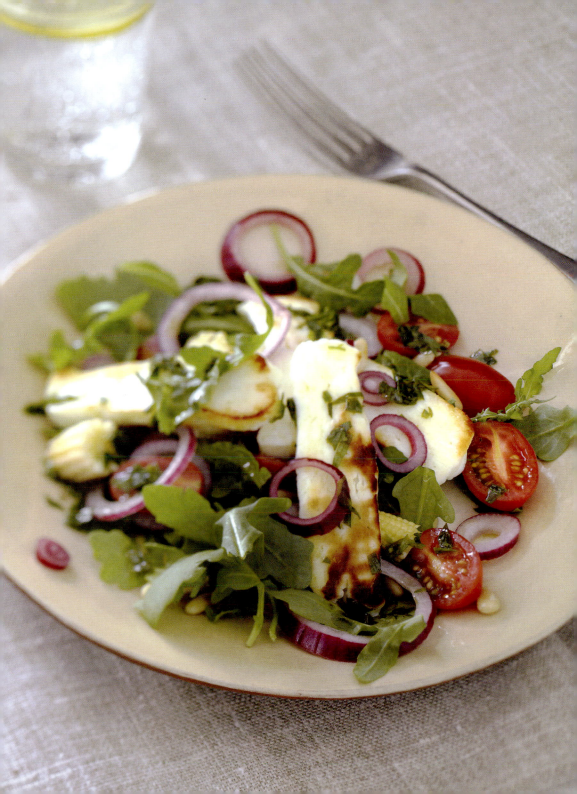

Yoghurt

Although generally thought of as a healthy product, it is only natural (plain), unsweetened yoghurt that is suitable for this eating plan. It is most often thought of as a protein-rich food, but it is also a notable source of carbohydrates. So it's always worth adding another source of protein to balance both food groups.

Yoghurt is a useful ingredient in marinades, as its inherent acid content naturally tenderises meat, and it can also be stirred into sauces instead of cream once the sauce is off the heat and has cooled slightly. But perhaps it is most useful as an instant, yet delicious, breakfast or snack if you add chopped fruit, nuts, or seeds.

All yoghurt naturally contains beneficial bacteria, or probiotics, and is therefore 'live'. Look for natural unsweetened yoghurt and ignore special labels of 'live yoghurt', which are meaningless. Flavoured yoghurts – even those that are low in fat and enriched with beneficial bacteria – contain sugar and should be avoided.

Three simple cooking techniques

As a dip Blend yoghurt with flavours of your choice: crushed garlic and chopped fresh dill; onion powder, grated onion, or chopped spring onion and grated cheese; fresh or dried chilli and chopped pimiento; deseeded diced cucumber and chopped fresh or dried mint. Season and chill until ready to serve with potato wedges, crudités, crackers, grilled meats, or fish.

As a lamb or chicken curry sauce Fry a chopped onion in a little sunflower oil. Blend some curry paste with natural unsweetened yoghurt and seasoning and add to the pan with some cooked diced lamb or chicken. Cook, stirring occasionally, for about 20 minutes until the yoghurt curdles, and then gradually the whey evaporates to leave a dryish sauce.

As a marinade or dressing As a marinade: blend yoghurt with a splash of olive or sunflower oil, season, and add flavours such as cumin, paprika, lemon juice, and chopped fresh coriander or dried chilli flakes, garlic, and the zest and juice of a lime. Use to marinate diced chicken, pork, lamb, or fish for 1–3 hours before grilling. Brush the remaining marinade over the food during cooking. As a dressing: blend yoghurt with a spoonful of crumbled blue or feta cheese and chopped fresh dill. Thin to the desired consistency with milk.

Meal suggestions

▶ Tandoori chicken: slash chicken breasts or skinned thigh or quarter portions with a knife. Marinate in natural unsweetened yoghurt with a spoonful or two of tandoori paste for at least 2 hours. Drain, place on the grill rack, and grill until cooked through and slightly charred in places. Serve with a vegetable curry and a salad (for lunch, add some chapattis).

▶ Yoghurt and prawn avocados: blend natural unsweetened yoghurt with some tomato purée and a splash of Worcestershire sauce. Add cooked peeled prawns. Pile onto halved, stoned avocados. Serve with green salad (for lunch, add brown bread).

▶ Natural whole milk or Greek-style yoghurt, crushed garlic, chopped fresh oregano, and a squeeze of lemon juice stirred into warm drained flageolet beans, topped with grated Parmesan or other Italian hard cheese (for lunch, spoon onto wholewheat pasta)

▶ Griddled halved tomatoes and aubergine slices, topped with Greek-style natural yoghurt mixed with crushed garlic, chopped, skinned, and deseeded cucumber, chopped mint, and seasoning, and sprinkled with toasted pine nuts (for lunch, add some couscous)

▶ Cooked ratatouille mixed with some drained canned haricot beans, topped with natural unsweetened yoghurt beaten with two eggs and some grated Cheddar cheese, and then baked until golden and set (for lunch, add warm wholewheat pittas)

Snack suggestions

▶ A spoonful or two of cooked leftover rice with some cooked peas, topped with natural unsweetened yoghurt flavoured with a dash of curry paste

▶ A spoonful of cooked puy or brown lentils mixed with a little natural unsweetened yoghurt and feta cheese dressing (bottom left), some sliced olives and chopped tomatoes in half a wholewheat pitta

▶ A small portion of yoghurt dip (opposite) with crudités

▶ Yoghurt and tomato smoothie: whizz some natural unsweetened yoghurt in a blender with canned tomatoes, a dash of Tabasco (or chilli powder) and some Worcestershire sauce. Serve with celery sticks.

What to look for
•Low-fat or fat-free cows milk, sheeps milk or goats milk natural unsweetened yoghurt
•Full-fat or whole milk cows milk, sheeps milk, or goats milk yoghurt (use occasionally)
•Soya yoghurts (the majority contain added sugar so you may have to shop around to find a sugar-free brand)
•Greek yoghurt is made by straining the yoghurt to remove the whey and give a thicker consistency. It is useful for cooking or making sauces, but be aware that some brands contain added cream and so should be used sparingly.

Ways to cook or serve
•Dip
•To enrich soups, sauces or stews
•Curry sauce
•Marinade
•Dressing

Simple ways to flavour
•Spices: chilli and cumin
•Herbs: fresh oregano, mint, dill, and thyme
•A few strands of saffron and a little crushed garlic mixed with natural unsweetened yoghurt and left in the fridge overnight; serve with cooked or cold meat (especially chicken or lamb).
•Blend with mayonnaise and chopped herbs to make a lighter dressing for eggs, asparagus, or cold salmon.

Yoghurt, avocado, and cucumber dip

This makes a delicious light lunch with crunchy garlic pittas, but is also great in smaller portions served as an accompaniment to any spiced grilled meat, poultry, fish, or even halloumi cheese. Alternatively, have extra crudités instead.

Make 4 or more portions

2 large, just ripe, avocados
Finely grated zest of 1 lime
1 tsp lime juice
½ cucumber

200ml natural unsweetened yoghurt
2 tbsp chopped fresh coriander
1 tbsp caraway seeds (optional)
Freshly ground black pepper

To serve: crudités – a selection of raw vegetables such as cherry tomatoes, radishes, and mangetout, or sticks of celery, carrot, courgette, and pepper

1. Halve the avocados, remove the stones, and scoop the flesh into a bowl, scraping the skin well to remove any flesh that has adhered to it. Mash thoroughly with a fork, adding the lime zest and juice as you do so.
2. Peel the cucumber and scoop out the seeds, then coarsely grate into a separate bowl. Squeeze to remove the excess moisture and pour it away. Add the cucumber to the avocado mix.
3. Beat in the yoghurt, coriander, and caraway seeds, then add a good grinding of black pepper. Cover and chill until ready to serve with plenty of crudités.

Lunch only
Serve with crunchy garlic pitta breads.
For the pittas:
1 large garlic clove, crushed
4 tbsp olive oil
4 wholemeal pitta breads
1 tbsp caraway seeds
A good pinch of coarse sea salt
To make the pittas, preheat the oven to 200°C (Gas 6). Put the crushed garlic in a small bowl and work in the olive oil. Split the pittas in half to make 8 thin ovals. Brush the garlic oil all over the crumbly sides of the pittas and sprinkle evenly with the caraway seeds and just a few grains of coarse sea salt. Cut each into 3 strips. Place on one large or two smaller baking sheets. Bake towards the top of the oven for 10–12 minutes until crisp and golden. Serve while still warm with the dip and crudités. Can be stored in an airtight container for several days.

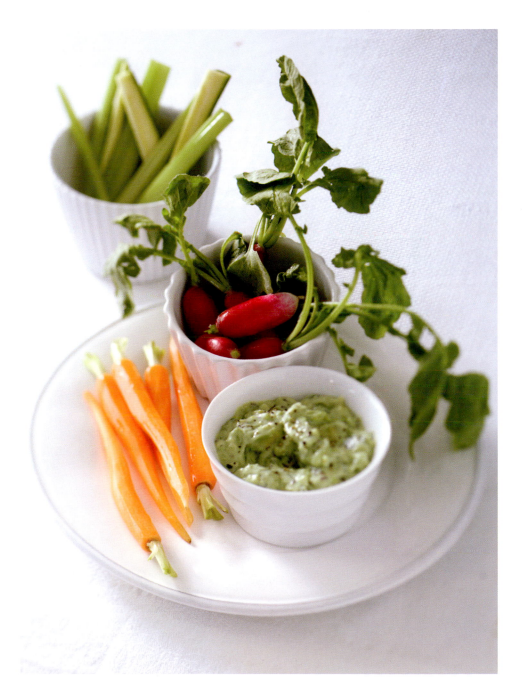

Chick-peas

Also known as garbanzos, chick-peas belong to the legume family and, like other vegetable-based proteins, they don't contain all the amino acids to qualify as 'complete'. They therefore need to be combined with other vegetable proteins to achieve a complete array of amino acids.

Chick-peas contain protein and carbohydrates, and are low in fat. They are wonderfully versatile and inexpensive to buy, either dried to be cooked or ready-cooked in cans. The dried beans need to be soaked in cold water for several hours or overnight (however, you can speed the soaking process by soaking them in boiling water for about 3 hours, then draining and cooking them as normal). To cook the soaked beans, boil them rapidly for 10 minutes to remove any toxins, then reduce the heat and simmer gently for 1–11/2 hours until they are really tender (115g of dried chick-peas, once soaked and cooked, are equivalent to a 410g can of ready-cooked chick-peas, drained).

Three simple cooking techniques

Roast Dry some cooked chick-peas on kitchen paper and tip into a bowl. Add a splash of olive oil and sprinkle with a pinch of chilli powder, cumin, and ground cinnamon (or use garam masala) and a little salt, if you like. Toss well and spread out on a baking tray. Roast in the oven at 230°C (Gas 8) for about 30 minutes, shaking the tray occasionally until they are crisp and brown. Leave to cool on the tray, then store in an airtight container.

Purée For houmous, tip cooked chick-peas or a drained can of chick-peas into a blender. Add a crushed garlic clove, a heaped tablespoonful of tahini paste, a good squeeze of lemon juice, and 2 tablespoons of olive oil. Blend until you have a thick, smooth paste. Season to taste and sharpen with more lemon juice if you like. Store in the fridge in an airtight container for up to 5 days.

Fried as falafel Put 2 drained cans of chick-peas in a processor with 1/2 a small chopped onion, a crushed garlic clove, 1/4 teaspoon chilli powder, 1 teaspoon ground cumin, 1 teaspoon ground turmeric, 1/2 teaspoon ground cinnamon, a small handful of parsley, the juice of a lemon, and salt and pepper. Process to a coarse paste. With wet hands, shape into small balls. Chill to firm. Fry in a little oil until golden on both sides. Drain on kitchen paper. Serve hot or cold.

Meal suggestions

▶ Chick-pea stew with garlic, tomatoes, mixed peppers, and fresh basil thrown in, and topped with grated mozzarella (for lunch, serve spooned over brown rice)

▶ Chick-pea, carrot, and mushroom curry, topped with a spoonful of natural unsweetened yoghurt and some toasted coconut Serve with a green salad (for lunch, add wholewheat chapattis)

▶ Felafel (left) served with salad and minted natural unsweetened yoghurt (for lunch, pack them into split wholewheat pitta breads with the salad and yoghurt)

▶ Chick-pea salad: mix cold cooked chick-peas with diced beetroot, cucumber, celery, and halved cherry tomatoes. Sprinkle with a little curry powder, lemon juice and sunflower oil and a large handful of chopped fresh coriander. Season and toss. Pile onto salad leaves and sprinkle with sunflower seeds (for lunch, add some cold cooked couscous).

▶ Harira (Moroccan soup): add a drained can of cooked chick-peas and a can of cooked green lentils to some stock with browned onions, skinned chicken thighs, garlic, ground cumin, ground coriander, chopped tomatoes, tomato purée, and a spoonful of harissa paste (which can have a fiery heat) and simmer. Take the chicken off the bones and return to the pot. Add a squeeze of lemon. Top with chopped fresh coriander (for lunch, serve with wholewheat Mediterranean flatbreads).

Snack suggestions

▶ A handful of roasted chick-peas (left). Eat with salad leaves

▶ Houmous (home-made, opposite, or bought) spread on 2 oatcakes, a piece of bread or toast, or eaten with some crudités

▶ 2 cold falafel and some cucumber slices

What to look for
• Dried (If you buy dried chick-peas, lentils, or beans, it's worth cooking a larger quantity, then freezing them in smaller portions to take out as required)
• Canned (in water with no added sugar or salt)

Ways to cook and serve
• Soup
• Stew or casserole
• Purée
• Cold in salads
• Roast
• Fried as falafel

Simple ways to flavour
• Spices: chilli, cumin, paprika
• With peppers and tomatoes in soups and stews
• Crushed with fresh coriander, lemon juice, and garlic as a side dish

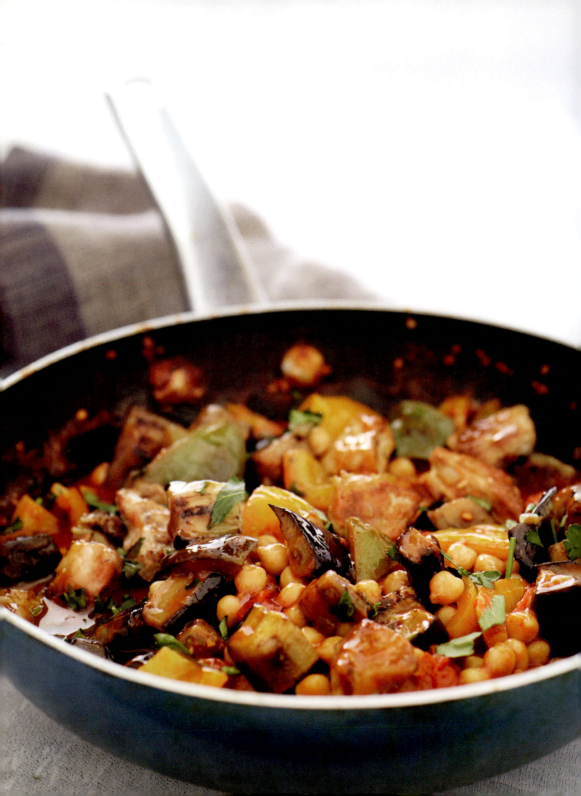

Chick-pea, pork, and aubergine ragout

This is a wonderful rich, hearty dish. You can also make a vegetarian version by omitting the pork and doubling the quantity of chick-peas. Add an extra splash of vegetarian Worcestershire sauce for flavour, if you wish.

Makes 4 portions

2 tbsp olive oil
1 large onion, chopped
225g diced pork, trimmed of all fat
2 small aubergines, diced
1 yellow pepper, diced
1 green pepper, diced
1 garlic clove, crushed
1 tsp smoked paprika
1 tbsp sweet paprika
1 x 400g can chopped tomatoes

2 tbsp tomato purée
150ml chicken or vegetable stock
2 x 410g cans chick-peas in water, drained (or 450g cooked [225g raw weight] chick-peas)
1 bay leaf
Freshly ground black pepper
2 tbsp chopped fresh parsley
4 tsp natural yoghurt, to garnish

To serve: a green salad

1. Heat the oil in a large, deep, non-stick frying pan or saucepan. Add the onion and fry, stirring, for 2 minutes to soften. Add the pork and brown, stirring and turning, for 2 minutes. Add the aubergines and peppers and cook, stirring, for 2 minutes.
2. Stir in the garlic and the two types of paprika, then add the canned tomatoes, tomato purée, stock, chick-peas, bay leaf, and a good grinding of black pepper. Bring to the boil, reduce the heat, cover, and simmer very gently for 1½ hours, stirring occasionally, until the sauce is rich and thick and the pork is really tender. Discard the bay leaf.
3. Stir in most of the parsley, reserving a little for garnish. Taste and re-season if necessary.
4. Spoon the ragout into warm bowls and top with a spoonful of yoghurt and a sprinkling of the remaining parsley. Serve with a green salad.

Lunch only
Omit one of the cans of chick-peas and spoon the ragout onto 250g cooked wholewheat tagliatelle.

Lentils and split peas

Like chick-peas, lentils and split peas are legumes – also known as pulses. They are a cheap, delicious, and versatile way of adding vegetable protein and carbohydrates to your diet. All legumes can be used to make a little meat go a lot further, as well as being a great basic ingredient for different vegetarian dishes.

Red and puy lentils are the only pulses that do not require soaking before cooking. Green, brown, and puy lentils hold their shape even when thoroughly cooked, whereas split peas and red lentils cook to a pulp. Lentils and split peas should always be boiled in plenty of water until tender – usually for around 45–50 minutes. (red lentils take 25–30 minutes). Always season legumes after cooking. If cooking a large quantity to be used later, allow them to cool quickly and then store in the fridge; don't leave them out at room temperature to become cold, or bacteria may grow, which could cause food poisoning.

Three simple cooking techniques

Pea and ham soup Put a meaty ham bone in a pan with some soaked split peas, a quartered onion, 2 chopped carrots, and a bay leaf. Add plenty of water and some seasoning. Bring to the boil, reduce the heat, part-cover, and simmer gently for 2 hours, or until really tender and the meat falls off the bone. Lift out the ham bone and cut off all the meat. Discard the bay leaf. Purée the contents of the pan, then add the chopped meat. Taste and re-season.

Simple dhal Brown an onion and a chopped garlic clove in a little sunflower or groundnut oil. Add a teaspoon each of grated fresh ginger, ground turmeric, cumin, and garam masala and fry for 30 seconds. Add 175g of red lentils and 450ml of vegetable stock. Simmer, stirring occasionally, until thick and pulpy. Season to taste.

Lentil loaf Brown a large chopped onion. Add 2 drained cans of lentils and mash with a fork. Mix in a large handful of chopped nuts, a large handful of grated Edam cheese, a tablespoon of chopped fresh thyme (or a teaspoon of dried), some Worcestershire sauce, seasoning, and 2 beaten eggs. Spoon into a greased 450g loaf tin. Press down. Cover with foil and bake at 190°C (Gas 5) for about 45 minutes until firm. Cool slightly, turn out, and serve sliced.

Meal suggestions

▸ Warm lentil and vegetable salad: cook some brown, green, or puy lentils. Drain. Add a mixture of diced cooked vegetables (leeks, courgettes, roots, green beans) and some peas or sweetcorn. Add some olive oil, lemon juice, a pinch of chilli powder, and crushed garlic. Add some chopped fresh coriander or parsley, toss, and serve (for lunch, add wholegrain bread).

▸ Lentil loaf (opposite), sliced warm or cold with warm or cold passata spooned over, and some vegetables or a salad (for lunch, add some cooked new potatoes)

▸ Pea and ham soup and a mixed salad with some pumpkin seeds and French dressing (for lunch, add wholemeal rolls)

▸ Dhal (opposite) with paneer or diced Edam cheese and cooked cauliflower stirred in at the last moment, topped with chopped onion fried in a little sunflower or groundnut oil until golden then some cumin seeds thrown in and fried for 30 seconds. Serve with a green salad (for lunch, add wholewheat chapattis)

▸ Lentil and mushroom stir-fry: stir-fry some ready-prepared stir-fry vegetables. Throw in some sliced mushrooms and cooked lentils, and flavour with oyster sauce and soy sauce (for lunch, spoon over udon [brown rice] noodles).

Snack suggestions

▸ A spoonful of cooked lentils mashed with a little French dressing, spooned onto rice cakes

▸ A handful of cooked lentils mixed with some rocket and a chopped tomato

▸ Some pease pudding (from a can) flavoured with curry paste, spread on a wholewheat chapatti, topped with shredded lettuce and a squeeze of lemon, and rolled up

What to look for

•Red lentils: quicker to cook than others (about 25 minutes). Use for soups, to thicken stews, and for spicy dhals.

•Dried peas: use for soups and pease pudding (soaked split peas simmered in stock with chopped onion for several hours until thick and porridgy. Also available canned).

•Green and brown lentils: 'meatier' texture than others. Use for soups, casseroles, curries, loaves, and patties.

•Puy lentils: smaller than green or brown lentils with a more delicate flavour. Considered the most sophisticated pulse, and often used dressed as a base for everything from grilled fish to pheasant breasts

Ways to cook and serve

•Soup
•Stew, casserole, or curry
•Purée and dhal
•Loaves, rissoles, and patties (brown, green, and puy)
•Salad
•Stir-fry

Simple ways to flavour

•Mushrooms, onions, and all root vegetables
•Lemon juice, garlic, a pinch of chilli powder, and olive oil as a dressing for a lentil salad
•Cheese, particularly mild varieties such as feta, halloumi, goats, Edam, or paneer (Indian curd cheese)

Lentil, red pepper, and harissa soup

Red lentils are so useful because they don't require any soaking first. This soup is best puréed, but can be left chunky if you prefer. If you like a more fiery taste, increase the harissa paste to 1 tablespoon.

Makes 4–6 portions

3 tbsp olive oil
1 red onion, chopped
1 garlic clove, chopped
1 carrot, diced
¼ celeriac, diced
2 red peppers, halved, deseeded, and diced
1 tsp ground cumin

1 tsp ground cinnamon
2 tsp sweet paprika
2 tsp harissa paste
225g red lentils
1.2 litres vegetable stock
1 tbsp chopped fresh thyme, plus extra for garnish
Freshly ground black pepper

1. Heat 2 tbsp of the oil in a large saucepan. Add the onion, garlic, carrot, and celeriac and cook, stirring, for 2 minutes over a moderate heat until beginning to soften but not brown.
2. Add all the remaining ingredients. Bring to the boil, stirring, then reduce the heat, cover, and simmer gently for 30 minutes, stirring occasionally, until everything is really tender.
3. Purée the soup in a blender or food processor, return to the pan, and taste and re-season if necessary. Reheat, ladle into warm bowls, and garnish with a tiny drizzle of remaining olive oil and a sprinkling of fresh thyme.

Lunch only
Serve with warm wholemeal flatbreads (such as khobez) or pitta breads.

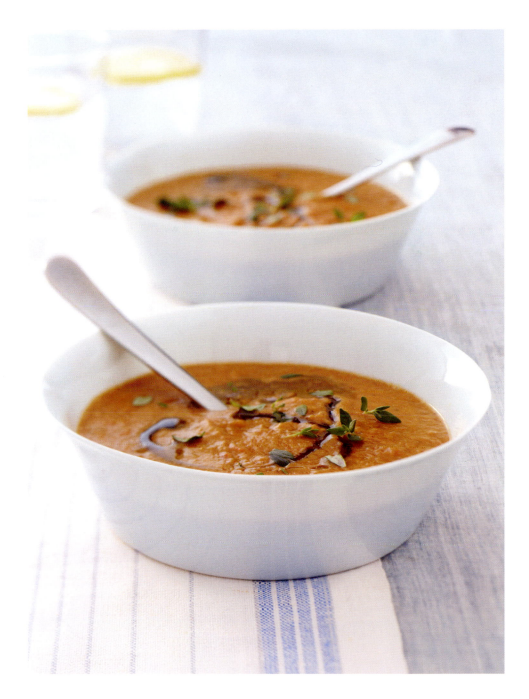

Dried beans

Dried beans This third group of the legume family ranges from large, plump butter beans, dried broad beans, deep red beans, and black beans to tiny green mung beans. They all add colour, flavour, and texture to a dish. As with chick-peas and lentils, they must be soaked for several hours first, then boiled rapidly for 10 minutes to remove toxins before simmering until tender (the time will depend on the bean; always follow instructions on the packet). Boil the beans until tender in water first before adding other flavourings (don't try to cook beans from raw in tomato juice, as the acid toughens the skins and prevents them becoming tender). If buying dried, always look for even-sized, shiny beans; those without a sheen will be old and of poor quality.

Canned beans in water are an excellent option. Keep a variety in your store-cupboard for quick, tasty meals. Canned baked beans in tomato sauce make a good snack and a quick meal option, but choose cans with no added sugar.

Three simple cooking techniques

Paté Purée cooked or drained canned beans with some garlic, lemon juice, and a little olive oil into a thick paste. Season and add some chopped celery, pepper, and cucumber.

Patties or rissoles Brown a finely chopped onion and garlic in a little oil. Put in a food processor with a can of drained butter or red kidney beans. Process briefly, scraping down the sides of the processor when necessary, until coarsely crushed (or put in a bowl and crush with the end of a rolling pin). Mix with some chopped nuts, Worcestershire sauce, soy sauce, and chopped fresh thyme. Season well. Mix with beaten egg to bind. Shape into little cakes or flattened balls. Chill for several hours. Fry in a non-stick frying pan with just a little sunflower oil until golden on both sides and cooked through.

Soup Brown an onion. Add other chopped vegetables of your choice, such as root vegetables, peppers, courgettes, and mushrooms. Add a can of any drained beans, a can of chopped tomatoes, some vegetable stock, and a bay leaf. Season and simmer until tender. Serve with grated cheese.

Meal suggestions

▸ Chilli beans: brown a chopped onion in a little sunflower oil. Add some cumin, chilli powder, and dried oregano. Stir in drained pinto or red kidney beans, a can of chopped tomatoes, and tomato purée. Season. Simmer until rich and thick. Serve with guacamole (p.183) (for lunch, add some corn tortillas).

▸ Warm flageolet and avocado salad with soft poached eggs: heat a can of flageolet beans in their liquid. Drain and add some chopped spring onions, lemon juice, and black pepper. Add a diced avocado and some baby leaf spinach. Toss gently, pile on plates, and top with soft poached eggs (p.42) (for lunch, add some cooked, still warm, baby new potatoes).

▸ Chilli con carne (try it with pinto beans instead of red kidney), topped with pickled jalapeño peppers, grated Cheddar cheese, and some shredded lettuce (for lunch, spoon over brown rice)

▸ Bean salad: drained white beans mixed with either tomatoes, garlic, onions, olives, and basil, and dressed with a little French dressing, or chopped radishes, tomatoes, cucumber, celery, and plenty of chopped fresh thyme and parsley, dressed in mayonnaise thinned with olive oil and white balsamic, and piled onto lettuce leaves (for lunch, add wholegrain bread)

▸ Bean rissoles (left) on a bed of wilted spinach with some warm passata spooned over and baby carrots (for lunch, add some potato wedges (pp.144–45), or a jacket potato)

Snack suggestions

▸ Nachos: crush red kidney beans, flavour with chilli and tomato purée, and spread on plain corn tortilla chips in a shallow ovenproof dish. Cover with some grated cheese. Bake at 190°C (Gas 5) until the cheese melts and the edges of the tortillas are crisp (if at work, just dip tortillas in the crushed bean mix)

▸ A little bean pâté spread on a wholewheat tortilla with some shredded lettuce and rolled up into a wrap

▸ A handful of soy nuts and an apple (soya 'nuts', which are, in fact, roasted soy beans, are crisp and lightly salted, and an excellent low-fat alternative to regular nuts)

What to look for
•Red kidney beans: robust and sweet. Use for chilli con carne, chilli beans, pâté, and salads.
•Black beans and mung beans: popular in Asian dishes
•Flageolet: pale green and creamy. Use in salads, soups, stews, casseroles, and as a side dish.
•Pinto beans: use for Mexican refried beans and chilli dishes
•Haricot, cannellini, black-eye, borlotti, and white kidney beans: soft and creamy. Use for baked beans and in salads, soups, stews, casseroles, and dips
•Butter and broad (fava) beans: sweet, floury-textured. Use as a side dish, dip, pâté, or in patties, rissoles, or curry.
•Soy beans: small and rich. Use for loaves and patties, rissoles, or burgers, in soups, stews, and casseroles (see also tofu and other soy products).

Ways to cook or serve
•Salads
•Soups, stews, and casseroles
•Pâtés and dips
•Loaves, patties, rissoles, burgers
•Curries and chillies
•Stir-fries

Simple ways to flavour
•Herbs: fresh thyme, rosemary, sage, and coriander
•Fresh and dried chillies
•Garlic and lemon or lime zest simmered with beans to serve as a side dish

Two-bean stew with shredded greens

This is based on a Middle Eastern soup, with the subtle spices complementing the vegetables, but it's more chunky and packed with nutrients. Use dried broad beans instead of butter beans or flageolet instead of black-eyed beans if you wish.

Makes 4 portions

2 tbsp olive oil
1 bunch of spring onions, chopped
2 garlic cloves, chopped
1 tsp ground turmeric
1 tsp ground cumin
¼ tsp ground cloves
750ml strong vegetable or
    chicken stock
1 x 410g can butter beans, drained
    (or 240g cooked [115g raw
    weight] beans)
1 x 410g can black-eyed beans, drained
    (or 240g cooked [115g raw
    weight] beans)

1 large turnip, diced
1 bay leaf
Freshly ground black pepper
125g spring greens or kale, finely
    shredded (discard the thick stumps)
2 courgettes, cut into thin ribbons with
    a potato peeler
2 tbsp chopped fresh parsley
2 tbsp chopped fresh coriander
2 tbsp tahini paste
150ml half-fat crème fraîche
A dash of lime juice

1. Heat the oil in a large saucepan. Add the spring onions and fry, stirring, for 1 minute. Add the garlic, turmeric, cumin, and cloves and fry for 30 seconds. Stir in the stock, beans, and turnip. Add the bay leaf and a good grinding of black pepper. Bring to the boil, reduce the heat, part-cover, and simmer gently for 15 minutes.
2. Add the greens and courgettes, stir, bring back to the boil, reduce the heat, cover, and simmer, stirring gently occasionally, for a further 8 minutes until everything is really tender. Discard the bay leaf.
3. Stir in the herbs, tahini paste, and all but 4 tsp of the crème fraîche (reserve the rest as a garnish). Sharpen to taste with lime juice and re-season if necessary.
4. Ladle into warm bowls and top each portion with a small dollop of the reserved crème fraîche.

Lunch only
Omit the courgettes and substitute 2 nests (100g) of wholewheat Chinese noodles when you add the greens in step 2.

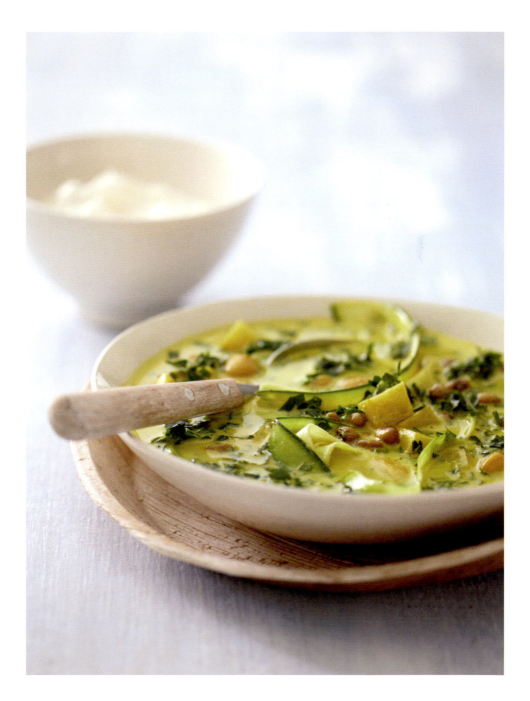

Nuts

Eating nuts is an excellent way to add protein to a meal or snack. Nuts are also a source of fats – particularly omega 6 fats, although some, such as walnuts, contain omega 3 fats, too – so they should be used to boost the protein level of a meal or snack rather than as a primary protein source for a main dish.

Always buy nuts in their unadulterated form – not honey-roasted, dry-roasted, or with another flavour – and always unsalted. Nuts that have been roasted or toasted will have been exposed to heat, which damages the sensitive fats they contain. It's best to buy the raw ingredients and cook them yourself to ensure that the temperature remains relatively low (below).

If you buy nut butter, choose whole-nut varieties where possible with no or minimal added salt, and avoid any containing sugar or palm oil. Peanut butter is the most familiar nut butter, but you should be able to find cashew, almond, macadamia, hazelnut, and mixed nut butters as well.

Three simple cooking techniques

Nut butter Warm 250g of your choice of nut in a saucepan, stirring for 2–3 minutes to release the oil slightly but not to toast them. Tip into a food processor and pulse into a smooth or chunky paste. Store in a clean screw-topped jar in the fridge and use within a couple of weeks.

To toast or roast To toast: heat a non-stick frying pan on a low heat, add nuts of your choice, and stir and shake the pan until they just turn golden. Tip out of the pan immediately to prevent burning. Scatter over a salad just before serving so they retain their crunch. To roast: toss mixed raw nuts in a little sunflower oil, then sprinkle with garam masala and a pinch of chilli powder (optional) and toss until well coated. Spread out in a roasting tin and roast at 150°C (Gas 2) for 30 minutes, or until browned, stirring and turning occasionally. Sprinkle with a few grains of coarse sea salt (if required) and serve warm or cool. Store in an airtight container for up to 2 weeks.

Vanilla nuts Fill a clean screw-topped jar with sweet nuts such as hazelnuts, pecans, cashews, and flaked almonds and a split vanilla pod. Leave at room temperature for at least 72 hours (shake the jar every 12 hours or so). Serve with yoghurt for a sweeter-tasting snack or after a main meal.

Meal suggestions

- Lentil and coconut curry: brown onions and mushrooms with curry paste, cooked lentils, stock, and some coconut cream. Simmer until rich and thick. Season and add chopped fresh coriander. Serve with lemon to squeeze over and a crisp green salad (for lunch, add brown basmati rice or chapattis).
- Peanut soup: soften finely chopped onion, carrot, and swede in a little sunflower oil. Add 1/2 jar whole-nut peanut butter, a pinch of chilli powder, and dried mixed herbs. Add some vegetable stock to give a thin but creamy consistency, then simmer until tender. Enrich with 1–2 tbsp reduced-fat crème fraîche. Serve topped with grated cheese. (For lunch, add wholegrain bread).
- Cashew quinoa paella: cook quinoa in stock with a pinch of saffron, browned chopped spring onions, red pepper and sliced mushrooms, a handful of frozen peas and some raw cashews. Serve with a green salad. (For lunch serve with some wholemeal bread).
- Chicken and mushroom skewers with satay sauce: thread cubes of chicken and button mushrooms on kebab skewers, brush with oil, sprinkle with caraway seeds and freshly ground black pepper, and grill. For the sauce, heat peanut butter and chilli powder, thinned with milk, stirring until smooth and thick, then seasoned to taste. Serve on a bed of wilted spinach with the sauce spooned over (for lunch, add some brown basmati rice).
- Chestnut and beef stew: make a beef stew with a little less beef and add a can or vacuum pack of cooked chestnuts. Once cooked, stir in 1–2 tbsp of thick, Greek-style yoghurt (for lunch, serve spooned over sweet potato mash).

Snack suggestions

- Nut butter of your choice spread on 2 rice cakes and topped with some sliced cucumber
- 2 spoonfuls of ground almonds blended into a vegetable smoothie with cooked carrots, tomato juice, and some chopped fresh basil, served with half a wholewheat bagel (optional)
- A small tub of plain, low-fat cottage cheese with a handful of chopped peanuts and some chopped pepper
- A handful of walnuts or pecans and a fresh pear

Protein

What to look for
- Walnuts, hazelnuts/cobnuts, chestnuts, almonds, pecans, Brazils, cashews, pistachios, macadamias, pine nuts, coconut and peanuts (although peanuts are technically legumes)

Note: Fresh nuts should be stored in an airtight container in a cool, dark place and used within a few weeks as, due to their high fat content, they can go rancid.

Ways to cook or serve
- Nut butter
- Toasted in salads
- Raw in curries and rice and pasta dishes
- Roasted flavoured nuts as a snack (opposite)
- Vanilla nuts for desserts or snacks (opposite)

Simple ways to flavour
- Cashews peanuts, coconut, and almonds all go well with curries and other hot, spicy dishes
- Pistachios, Brazils, chestnuts, and macadamias are best with more delicate flavours such as chicken, fish, and veal. They also go well with sweet spices such as cinnamon and star anise.
- Walnuts, pecans, almonds, pine nuts, and hazelnuts are particularly good with cheeses and in salads and with sweet herbs like rosemary, coriander, parsley, or basil for pesto.

Rosemary, garlic, and almond pesto

Flavour chicken, lamb, oily fish, or pork before grilling with this pesto, and serve with a large mixed salad. Or thin it with a little oil to make a salad dressing for a salad with flageolet beans.

Makes 8 or more portions

4 large fresh rosemary sprigs
   (about 15g)
1 bunch of fresh parsley (about 30g)
2 large garlic cloves, lightly crushed
55g ground almonds

A good grinding of black pepper
55g freshly grated Parmesan or other
   Italian hard cheese
6 tbsp olive oil

To serve: extra Parmesan or other
Italian hard cheese and a mixed salad

1. Pull the leaves from the woody rosemary stems. Discard the stems.
2. Put the rosemary leaves and all the parsley (including the stalks) in a food processor with the garlic, almonds, black pepper, cheese, and 4 tbsp of the oil. Process well until blended, stopping and scraping down the sides of the processor as necessary.
3. With the machine still running, gradually add the remaining oil until you have a shiny paste. (Alternatively, pound the herbs and garlic in a mortar with a pestle. Gradually add the nuts, working them to a paste with the herbs. Add the pepper, then work in a little of the cheese, then a little of the oil and continue until both are used up.) Add 2 tbsp boiling water and blend again or stir in.
4. Store the remaining pesto in a clean jar in the fridge for up to 2 weeks, covered with an extra spoonful of olive oil to keep the air out.

Lunch only
Serve mixed with wholewheat spaghetti.
For 4 portions, cook 350g of spaghetti according to the packet directions. Drain and return to the pan. Add half the pesto and toss gently so every strand is coated. Pile on warm plates or in bowls and serve with extra Parmesan (or other Italian hard cheese) and a mixed salad.

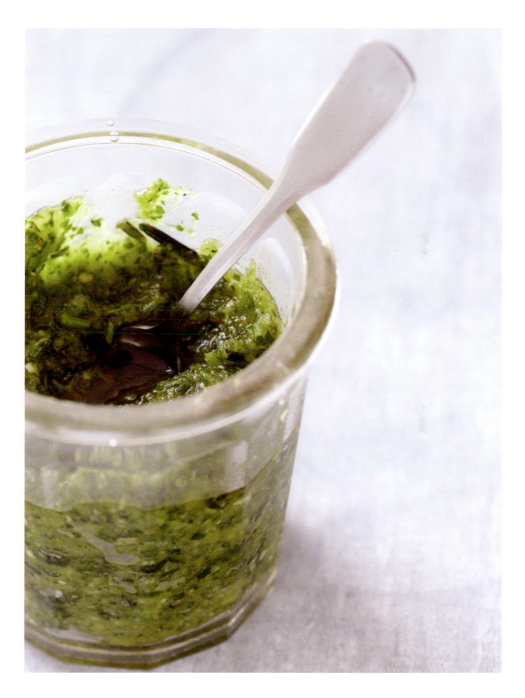

Quinoa

Quinoa is treated like a grain, although it technically qualifies as a seed. Some people pronounce it 'keen-waa', which the traditional South American way of saying it, while others use the more anglicised version, 'kwin-oh-aa'. As it is a seed, it also contains some fat, although it is predominantly a source of complex (rather than refined) carbohydrates.

Unlike most grains, quinoa is also a worthy source of protein, as it has the full complement of amino acids. This makes it a rare grain-based complete protein. Because of this high protein content, it can be eaten in the evenings if you want a more substantial meal.

Once boiled or steamed, cool the quinoa quickly if you are not eating immediately and store it in the fridge; like rice and legumes, it can harbour bacteria if left at room temperature for a long period.

Three simple cooking techniques

Steam Use 1 part quinoa to 2 parts lightly salted water or stock. Put the quinoa in a pan, add the boiling water or stock, bring back to the boil, stir well, cover, reduce the heat, and simmer for about 15 minutes, or until the liquid is absorbed and the seeds have little 'tails'. Remove from the heat and leave to stand for 5 minutes, then fluff up with a fork.

Toast Heat a large non-stick frying pan. Add some dry quinoa and toast, stirring and turning until golden and starting to pop, then tip into a bowl. Store in sealed container in the fridge and use as a dry cereal, or steam in the usual way (it gives it a lovely nutty flavour).

Salad Steam some quinoa and spread it out on a plate to cool quickly, then tip into a bowl. Add chopped peppers, tomatoes, cucumber, radishes, some fresh raw, or drained, canned (in water) sweetcorn kernels. Add some chopped walnuts. Toss the ingredients in a dressing made with olive oil, a splash of walnut oil, white balsamic, and plenty of fresh black pepper.

Meal suggestions

▸ Quinoa and chick-pea salad: steam, cool, and mix the quinoa with cooked chick-peas, chopped fresh coriander, some chopped spring onions, red pepper, and sun-kissed tomatoes. Dress with olive oil, a splash of red-wine vinegar, and plenty of black pepper (for lunch, add some wholegrain bread).

▸ Quinoa and butternut squash pilaf: steam in stock with cubes of butternut squash, diced carrots, chopped fresh thyme, and chopped spring onions. Sprinkle with toasted pumpkin seeds and crumbled feta cheese (for lunch, add some rolled-up wholewheat tortillas).

▸ Quinoa and vegetable stew: brown an onion in some olive oil. Add 1 part quinoa and 3 parts stock and diced vegetables of your choice. Add a bouquet garni and seasoning. Simmer for 20–30 minutes, or until all the vegetables are tender. Discard the bouquet garni and re-season if necessary. Serve sprinkled with grated Cheddar or Edam cheese (for lunch, add some potatoes to the stew).

▸ Prawn and saffron quinoa: steam quinoa in stock (opposite), but add some saffron strands to the stock. After 5 minutes, add some raw king prawns, some sliced mushrooms, and some thawed frozen peas. Leave to stand for 5 minutes, fluff up, and serve with lemon wedges to squeeze over and a watercress salad (for lunch, add some wholewheat pittas).

▸ Mushroom quinoa pilaf: brown an onion in a little olive oil and add some sliced mushrooms and some fresh chopped thyme. Stir in 1 part quinoa and 2 parts stock, steam (opposite), leave to stand 5 minutes, fluff up, and serve with Parmesan (or other Italian hard cheese) shavings and a green salad (for lunch, add some wholewheat chapattis).

Snack suggestions

▸ A handful of sprouted seeds, a few cherry tomatoes, chopped fresh parsley, and a drizzle of French dressing mixed into 2 spoonfuls of cold leftover quinoa

▸ A spoonful of toasted quinoa cereal with a chopped apple

▸ 2 spoonfuls of leftover quinoa and chick-pea salad (above)

What to look for

• Quinoa can be bought 'dry' and should be cooked in the same way that one might prepare rice, perhaps using vegetable or chicken stock to add flavour. Ready-cooked quinoa is becoming increasingly popular and can be eaten straight from the packet without refrigeration (it must be kept in the fridge after opening).

Ways to cook or serve

• Steam
• Salad
• Stir-fry
• Soups, stews, and casseroles
• Sprout for salads and snacks (see bean sprouts, pp.184–85)
• Toast

Simple ways to flavour

• For a salad or accompaniment instead of bulgur wheat, with fresh herbs, garlic oil, and some lemon juice
• As a side dish instead of couscous with chopped nuts and seeds and grated orange or lime zest
• Cooked with coconut milk or tomato juice and a bay leaf and half the amount of stock as a base for a pilaf
• Drizzled with truffle oil or walnut oil to enhance its nutty flavour

Curried quinoa and vegetable pilaf with toasted coconut

This is a complete meal that needs no accompaniment except chapattis, if serving at lunchtime. Substitute other vegetables of your choice, such as any winter or summer squash, broad beans, peppers, or celeriac, if you wish.

Makes 4 portions

2 tbsp sunflower oil
1 onion, chopped
2 tbsp mild curry paste
300g quinoa
1 large carrot, finely diced
1 turnip or ¼ swede, finely diced
1 x 400ml can coconut milk

400ml vegetable stock
Freshly ground black pepper
30g coconut flakes
1 courgette, finely diced
55g French beans, cut in short lengths
55g fresh shelled or frozen peas
A few torn coriander leaves

1. Heat the oil in a large saucepan or wok. Add the onion and stir for 3 minutes until lightly golden. Stir in the curry paste and cook for 30 seconds.
2. Stir in the quinoa until coated in the oil and curry paste. Add the quinoa, carrot, turnip, coconut milk, and stock. Season. Bring to the boil, reduce the heat, stir, cover, and simmer gently for 12 minutes. Add the remaining vegetables, cover, and cook for a further 8 mintues, or until cooked through and most of the liquid has been absorbed. (The quinoa will have little white 'tails', too.) Taste and re-season, if necessary. Fluff up with a fork.
3. Meanwhile, toss the coconut in a hot non-stick frying pan for 2–3 minutes until lightly golden, then immediately tip out of the pan onto a plate so it doesn't burn.
4. Spoon the quinoa pilaf onto warm plates, top with the toasted coconut, and scatter a few torn coriander leaves over the top.

Lunch only
Serve with warm chapattis.

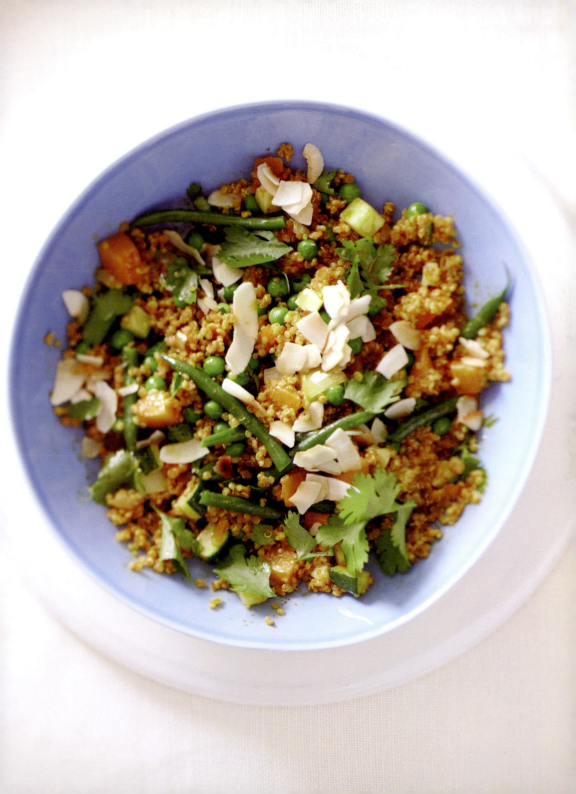

Quorn

A versatile and complete source of vegetarian protein, quorn is low in fat and calories yet high in fibre. Quorn is the brand name of a mycoprotein, a protein that is grown from a fungus (like mushrooms) and glucose, and then bound with egg white to provide a formed texture.

Because it has a very bland taste and absorbs flavours easily, quorn can take on just about any flavour you wish to marry with it, and is also good marinated before cooking. It is tender even when raw, so it is best not to overcook it. Quorn doesn't shrink on cooking so you need less of it – 350g of Quorn mince, unlike beef mince, for example, is plenty for four portions.

Quorn is available in the chiller cabinet or frozen (there is no need to defrost it before cooking). It can also be found in a variety of ready meals, ready-flavoured pieces, sausages, and burgers, but, as with other processed foods, these products are best avoided because of their high added sugar and salt content.

Three simple cooking techniques

Bolognese sauce Brown an onion and a crushed garlic clove in a little olive oil. Add some minced Quorn, a can of chopped tomatoes, tomato purée, a splash of apple juice, some dried oregano, and a bay leaf. Season. Simmer for about 10 minutes or until rich and thick, then discard the bay leaf.

Grill For barbecued Quorn steaks, mix a marinade of tomato purée, a splash of sunflower oil, white balsamic, soy sauce, and Worcestershire sauce in a shallow dish. Marinate the Quorn fillets for 30 minutes. Grill for 2–3 minutes on each side until golden, brushing the fillets with the leftover marinade every so often as they cook.

Stir-fry Heat a little sunflower oil in a large frying pan or wok. Add spring onions cut into short lengths, sliced peppers, mushrooms, tomatoes, and courgettes and stir-fry for 2 minutes. Add Quorn steak strips and stir-fry for 2–3 minutes. Add some Worcestershire sauce, seasoning, and a pinch of dried chilli flakes and toss well (for lunch, wrap in corn torillas).

Meal suggestions

▸ Quorn moussaka: make the bolognese mixture (opposite), but flavour with ground cinnamon, too. Layer with griddled aubergine or courgette slices. Top with natural unsweetened yoghurt beaten with an egg and some grated cheese. Bake at 190°C (Gas 5) until set and golden. Serve with a green salad (for lunch, add some wholewheat pitta breads).

▸ Fajitas (lunch only): stir-fry (left) and spoon onto corn or wholewheat tortillas. Add a dollop of half-fat crème fraîche, roll up, and serve with guacamole (p.183).

▸ Barbecued Quorn steaks with a large mixed salad (for lunch, add jacket potatoes topped with a dollop of half-fat crème fraîche and some chopped chives)

▸ Quorn and vegetable soup. Make a vegetable soup and add some minced Quorn for the last 10 minutes of cooking. Serve topped with grated cheese (for lunch, add wholegrain bread or a roll).

▸ Vegetable Bolognese: make the sauce (opposite). Pare strips of carrot and courgette with a potato peeler. Steam until tender. Pile on plates, top with the Quorn Bolognese sauce and some grated Parmesan (or other Italian hard cheese). Serve with a green salad (for lunch use wholewheat spaghetti instead of or as well as the vegetable ribbons).

Snack suggestions

▸ A spoonful of leftover stir-fry rolled in a lettuce leaf

▸ 1/2 cold barbecued Quorn fillet, sliced, on a large wholegrain cracker spread with a little mayonnaise and topped with some sliced cucumber

▸ Quorn bites: sauté some Quorn pieces in a splash of olive oil with some Cajun spices for 3–4 minutes until cooked through. Drain on kitchen paper, cool quickly, and store in the fridge. Have 4–5 chunks in half a wholewheat pitta with some shredded lettuce.

What to look for
•Beef- or chicken-style pieces: use instead of diced meat or poultry for any stew or casserole.
•Fillets: use instead of chicken breasts, pork lamb, beef, or venison steaks. (Don't be put off by their small size, they are quite filling.)
•Steak strips: use for stir-fries and fajitas.
•Mince: use in any dish that calls for mince.

Ways to cook or serve
•Bake (in a pie)
•Grill
•In a sauce, e.g, Bolognese
•Stir-fry or sauté
•Soup
•Stew, casserole or curry

Simple ways to flavour
•Ripe tomatoes, garlic, onions, and fresh torn basil for a Mediterranean flavour
•Chilli, cumin, and oregano for a more Mexican flavour
•Cinnamon, mint, coriander, and ginger for a Middle Eastern zing

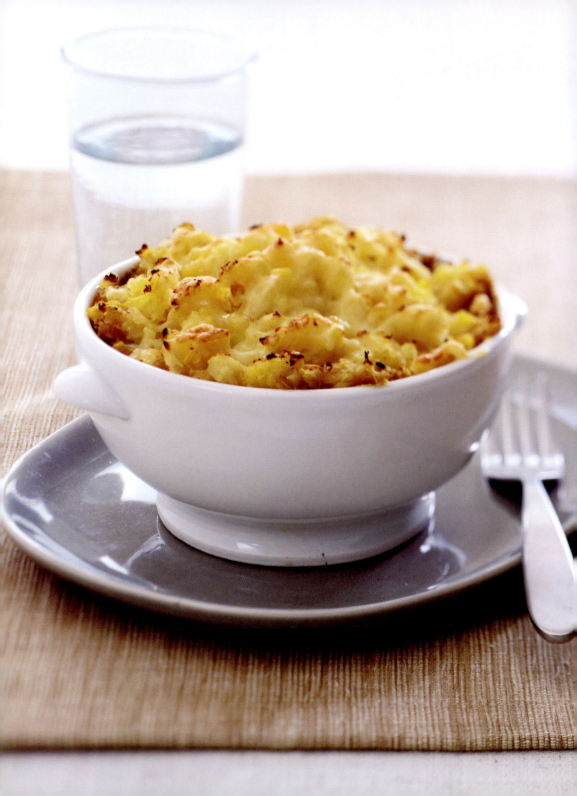

Quorn cottage pie

The advantage of Quorn is that it will take on any flavour you fancy. It is guaranteed to be tender, too, and makes a delicious nutritious meal even if you aren't vegetarian. Edam cheese doesn't melt as well as Cheddar, but it still makes an attractive, tasty topping, and is lower in fat.

Makes 4 portions

1 tbsp sunflower oil
1 onion, finely chopped
115g button mushrooms, sliced
¼ swede, finely diced or grated
2 carrots, finely diced or grated
55g shelled fresh or frozen peas
350g minced Quorn
½ tsp dried mixed herbs
600ml vegetable stock

To serve: leafy greens

1 tbsp tomato purée
1 tbsp soy sauce
Freshly ground black pepper
1 bay leaf
¾ swede (about 500g), peeled and cut into small chunks
1 celeriac (about 350g), peeled and cut into small chunks
A small knob of butter
A good pinch of grated nutmeg
55g Cheddar or Edam cheese, grated

1. Heat the oil in a large saucepan. Add the onion and fry, stirring for 3 minutes until lightly golden.
2. Add the mushrooms, swede, carrots, peas, Quorn, and herbs, then stir in the stock, tomato purée, soy sauce, and a good grinding of black pepper. Add the bay leaf. Bring to the boil, reduce the heat, cover and simmer gently for 20 minutes until the vegetables are tender. Turn up the heat and boil rapidly for about 2 minutes to reduce slightly and thicken the liquid.
3. Meanwhile, cook the swede and celeriac in boiling water with a pinch of salt added, if you like, for about 10 minutes, or until tender. Drain and return to the pan. Heat for a minute or 2, stirring, to dry out. Mash with the butter, nutmeg, and a good grinding of black pepper. Beat well with a wooden spoon until smooth.
4. Preheat the oven to 190°C (Gas 5). Spoon the mixture into a 1.2-litre shallow ovenproof dish or 4 individual dishes. Top with the celeriac mash and fluff it up with a fork. Sprinkle the cheese over the top. Bake in the oven for about 40 minutes until golden. Serve hot with some leafy greens.

Lunch only
Substitute 1 large sweet potato for the swede and 1 large potato for the celeriac.

Mixed seeds

One of the ultimate convenience foods, seeds are an instant way of adding protein to your meals and snacks. A couple of tablespoons of seeds scattered over a breakfast bowl of porridge, a handful eaten with an apple or pear mid-morning, or tossed into a mixed salad at lunchtime is ideal. They are also an excellent protein to combine with complex carbohydrates such as couscous, bulgur wheat, rice, and pasta as well as adding great texture and flavour to vegetables. Seeds also contain a certain amount of fat, but it's the longer-term energy they provide, rather than the calories they contain, that's important.

The most common seeds to buy are pumpkin, sesame, and sunflower seeds, and also linseeds (flaxseeds), which contain a lot of fibre. Other seeds can be used for flavouring, too, such as poppy, celery, cumin, coriander, and fennel seeds. Avoid tubs of seeds coated in a sweetened mix. Seeds are best scattered over food just before serving (so they don't become soggy), or added to roasting vegetables.

Three simple cooking techniques

Toast Heat a tablespoon or so of olive or sunflower oil in a non-stick frying pan. Add the seeds and toss over a gentle heat until puffed and browned. Tip into a bowl. Season with a little salt, if liked, and leave to cool. Store in a screw-topped jar.

Roast Preheat the oven to 150°C (Gas 2). Spread the seeds out on a baking tray. Drizzle with a little olive or sunflower oil and toss. Bake for about 15 minutes until they start to pop. Season as you like and tip onto kitchen paper to drain and cool. Store in a screw-topped jar.

Flavour seeds Although raw seeds have a pleasant nutty taste, you can add other savoury flavourings, such as a sprinkling of garam masala, Cajun spices, or cumin before toasting or roasting. Toss well.

Meal suggestions

- A large mixed salad with some cubed beetroot, a little crumbled feta cheese, and a few tablespoons of toasted pumpkin seeds
- Mixed roasted root vegetables with pumpkin and sunflower seeds added, and some fresh chopped thyme
- Mixed seeds stirred into cooked bulgur wheat with chopped fresh chilli and coriander, and spiked with lime juice
- Sesame seeds sprinkled over small scrubbed potatoes that have been tossed in a little olive oil and roasted until golden, and served with an avocado and mixed-leaf salad
- Mixed seeds and grated Parmesan (or other Italian hard cheese) sprinkled over wholewheat pasta with tomato sauce

Snack suggestions

- 1 small handful of seeds stirred into 1 small pot of natural unsweetened yoghurt
- 1 small handful of seeds and 1 apple or pear
- 1 small handful of seeds with a small fruit or vegetable smoothie
- 1 small handful of seeds and some leftover cold vegetables with a dash of soy sauce

What to look for
- Buy in separate packs or ready-mixed and store in jars in a cool, dark place.
- Buy in smallish quantities and use within a month or so, as they contain a lot of oil that will go rancid in time.
- Tubs of savoury-flavoured mixed seeds are another option for salads and snacks.

Ways to cook or serve
- Raw
- Toasted in a pan
- Roasted in the oven. You can toast and roast raw bought seeds (and you can buy them ready-toasted), but you can also use the scooped-out seeds of a pumpkin or other squash, and their flavour is far superior. Wash the scooped-out seeds well, remove any strings or bits of flesh, then pat them dry on kitchen paper.

Simple ways to flavour
- Spices: chilli, cumin, garam masala, cinnamon, Cajun spices, freshly ground black pepper
- With chopped nuts and cereals like rolled oats, wheat, barley, or millet flakes for breakfast

Salad of mixed seeds with roasted aubergine and crumbled feta cheese

Serve this flavoursome salad as an accompaniment to casseroles and tagines, grilled kebabs, chicken, fish, or steaks.

Makes 4 portions

2 aubergines
4 spring onions, finely chopped
2 tbsp fresh chopped parsley
2 tbsp chopped fresh mint
½ cucumber, diced
175g cherry tomatoes, halved
4 tbsp olive oil
1 large garlic clove, crushed

Finely grated zest and juice
  of ½ lemon
2 tbsp white balsamic
Freshly ground black pepper
2 tbsp each pumpkin, sunflower, and
  sesame seeds
115g feta cheese, crumbled
A few stoned black olives

1. Preheat the grill. Trim the stalks from the aubergines and discard. Put the aubergines in the grill pan and grill for 20 minutes, turning occasionally, until just soft. Do not allow to burn. Place them in a plastic bag and leave to cool, then cut them into bite-sized chunks.
2. Mix the aubergine chunks with the spring onions, parsley, mint, cucumber, and tomatoes. Whisk the oil, garlic, lemon zest and juice, and the white balsamic together. Pour over the salad, season with plenty of black pepper, and toss well.
3. Cover and chill for at least 2 hours in the fridge before serving to allow the flavours to develop. Pile into shallow bowls and scatter the seeds, feta, and olives over the top before serving.

Lunch only

Put 225g bulgur wheat in a large bowl. Add 600ml boiling vegetable stock, stir, and leave to stand for 30 minutes, or until swollen and soft and all the water has been absorbed. Make the rest of the dish while it's standing, then mix with the other ingredients and chill.

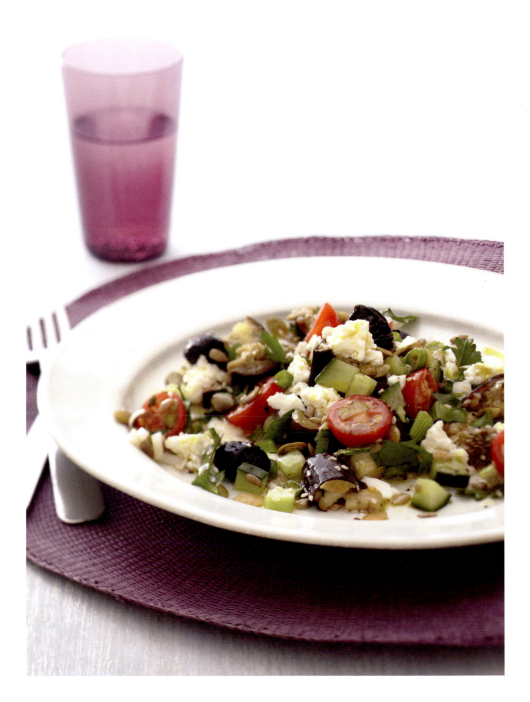

Soy products and tofu

Soy beans can be eaten fresh or dried. They are also ground down and mixed with water to make soy milk and yoghurt (p.63), made into curds and then pressed and cut into blocks to make tofu (bean curd), or turned into miso paste and powdered soup.

The bright-green fresh soy beans, also known as edamame beans, make great snacks, and the shelled green beans are a good alternative to baby broad beans. Soya beans are also used to make tempeh and soy sauce. They contain protein as well as carbohydrates and fat, making them almost a complete food in themselves. Miso paste is used as a soup base and in marinades. TVP (textured vegetable protein) is processed dried soya protein, which, when rehydrated, has the spongy texture of meat. It, too, is a high-quality protein. TVP mince makes an inexpensive alternative to minced meat (and you need only a third of the quantity compared with fresh meat. Just reconstitute with boiling water as directed on the packet).

Three simple cooking techniques

Stir-fry Marinade tofu cubes in soy sauce, lemon juice, chilli, ginger, and garlic. Heat a little oil in a large frying pan or wok. Stir-fry the drained cubes for 2–3 minutes. Sprinkle with any remaining marinade.

Curry Brown a chopped onion and some garlic in a little sunflower oil. Add Madras curry paste and fry for 30 seconds. Add cubed firm tofu, lightly steamed tempeh, or reconstituted TVP mince. Toss for 2 minutes. Add some stock or coconut milk and seasoning. Simmer for 15–20 minutes, or until thickened, then add chopped fresh coriander.

Miso soup Simmer finely chopped spring onions, carrots, and some sliced mushrooms in plenty of vegetable stock. Blend a spoonful of miso paste with a spoonful of water and stir it into the vegetables and stock.

Meal suggestions

▸ Tofu kedgeree (lunch only): fry an onion in a little sunflower oil, add diced smoked tofu and peas and stir-fry for a few minutes. Flavour with curry powder. Stir into freshly cooked brown rice and add quartered hard-boiled eggs. Toss until piping hot. Serve with a green salad.

▸ Green soya bean salad: mix cooked frozen soya beans with chopped spring onions, sliced raw mushrooms, halved cherry tomatoes, diced yellow pepper, and some pumpkin seeds. Toss in a dressing of olive oil, a little harissa paste, a splash of red-wine vinegar, and a little apple juice. Pile onto a bed of baby spinach (for lunch, add wholegrain bread).

▸ Tempeh or tofu kebabs: marinate cubes in soy sauce, chilli flakes, white balsamic, and some sunflower oil for at least 1 hour. Thread on skewers. Grill, brushing with more marinade, until golden, turning once. Serve with a large bean sprout, shredded Chinese leaf, and mixed shredded pepper salad tossed in oil, soy sauce, and apple juice (for lunch, add brown rice or cooked udon [brown rice] noodles to the salad)

▸ Curry: make as before (opposite), but add some cooked cauliflower florets and frozen peas for the last 5 minutes of cooking time. Serve with a green salad dressed with lime juice and sprinkled with toasted coconut (for lunch, spoon over brown basmati rice).

▸ Tempeh or tofu and peanut stir-fry: marinate and stir-fry as before (left), but add a handful of raw peanuts and some shredded pak choi and cucumber to the pan (for lunch, spoon over brown rice).

Snack suggestions

▸ Edamame pods with a little soy sauce to dip
▸ A spoonful of silken tofu in a fruit or vegetable smoothie
▸ Silken tofu with some chopped fresh pear

What to look for
• Tofu: sold as softer, creamier, silken tofu or a dense, firm block. Use silken for dips, sauces, spreads, and dressings. Use firm tofu as a meat substitute.
• Tempeh: a flat white cake with a mushroom-like flavour. Slice and fry until golden or use in soups, stews, and stir-fries.
• Edamame: buy frozen or fresh in their pods or shelled.
• Miso paste and soup: the paste is sold in jars, the soup in sachets.
• TVP: dried soya mince available alongside dried beans
• Soy sauce: sold as dark, light, or and reduced salt. Tamari is a Japanese dark soy sauce.

Ways to cook or serve
• Grill
• Bake
• Stir-fry or sauté
• Curry, casserole, or stew
• Dip or spread
• Marinade, sauce, or dressing
• Salad
• Soup

Simple ways to flavour
• Far Eastern flavours (for tofu, edamame, and tempeh): garlic, ginger, chilli, lemon grass, soy sauce, wasabi paste
• Middle Eastern flavours (for edamame): harissa paste, star anise, cinnamon, nutmeg, cloves
• Savoury (for silken tofu as a dip or dressing): chives, parlsey, mint, or coriander

Tofu and sugar snap pea green curry

Firm tofu will take good strong flavours, so it is excellent for a curry (or you could substitute Quorn, if you prefer). If serving it at lunchtime, substitute potatoes for the celeriac and add some brown long-grain rice.

Makes 4 portions

225g sugar snap peas
1 tbsp sunflower oil
4 spring onions, cut in short lengths
1 small celeriac, peeled and cut into
    walnut-sized pieces
2 tbsp Thai green curry paste

1 x 410g can coconut milk
1 tbsp Thai fish sauce
350g block firm tofu, dried on kitchen
    paper and cubed
2 tomatoes, quartered
A few torn fresh coriander or flat
    parsley leaves

1. Arrange the sugar snap peas in an even layer in a metal colander or steamer, cover, and steam for about 4 minutes until the peas are just tender but still have some 'bite'.
2. Heat the oil in a separate pan. Add the spring onions and fry, stirring for 2 minutes until lightly coloured. Add the celeriac and cook, stirring for 1 minute. Stir in the curry paste and coconut milk. Add the Thai fish sauce. Bring to the boil, reduce the heat, cover, and simmer, stirring occasionally, for 15 minutes, or until the celeriac is tender.
3. Add the tofu, cover, and simmer very gently for a further 10 minutes.
4 Stir the sugar snap peas into the curry and add the quartered tomatoes. Simmer for 2 minutes until the tomatoes are softened slightly but still hold their shape. Spoon the curry into bowls and scatter over a few torn fresh coriander or flat parsley leaves.

Lunch only
Serve with 225g sticky brown long-grain rice.
Put the rice in a pan with 750ml water. Bring to the boil, reduce the heat, cover, and simmer very gently for 40 minutes until the rice is tender and the water has been absorbed. The texture should be slightly sticky. Add 1 tsp Thai fish sauce to the rice and stir well. Spoon the sticky rice into bowls and top with the curry.

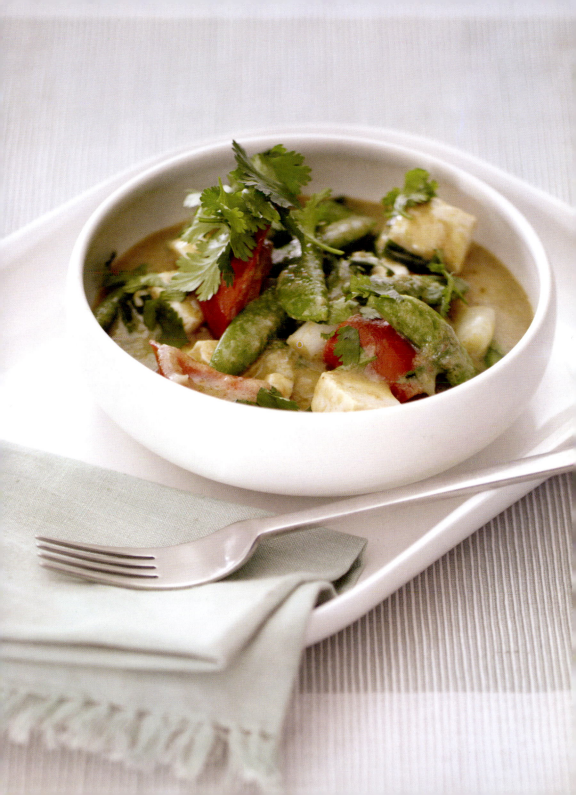

Mackerel, herring, sardines (pilchards)

These oily fish, with their dark flesh, are rich in omega-3 fats. Mackerel, which has a blue-green mottled skin, and shiny silver herring are inexpensive and make delicious eating hot or cold. They are also available smoked (herrings become known as kippers, bloaters, and buckling when smoked). Cornish sardines (which are really pilchards because they are slightly larger than sardines) are a good choice. Sprats and anchovies also fall into this category, but are not widely available fresh. Canned fish is an excellent store-cupboard standby and a good source of calcium if you eat the soft, cooked bones, so keep cans of sardines, pilchards, and mackerel in your kitchen. Anchovies, available either in salt or oil in jars or cans, are a wonderful addition to many hot and cold dishes.

Herrings and sardines need scaling before cooking. Rub the scales off with your thumb, then rinse the fish under cold water.

Three simple cooking techniques

Grill Clean the fish if necessary and scale herrings and sardines. Slash the flesh of the mackerel or herring several times with a sharp knife on either side before cooking. Brush lightly with sunflower or olive oil and season with freshly ground black pepper. Push some fresh herbs into the body cavity if you like. Grill for 5 minutes each side for whole mackerel or herring, 2–3 minutes each side for sardines or fillets.

Souse (herring or mackerel fillets) Remove any stray bones. Sprinkle the fillets with salt, leave for 5 minutes, then rinse and pat dry. Put some thinly sliced onion and chopped fresh dill on the flesh (not the skin side) and roll up. Pack in a shallow ovenproof dish. Cover with equal parts white balsamic and white-wine vinegar. Add some peppercorns and a bay leaf. Cover with foil and bake in the oven at 180°0C (Gas 4) for 45 minutes. Serve warm, or leave to cool in the liquid and then chill for 24 hours before serving.

Paté Use cooked smoked mackerel or drained canned fish. Put in a food processor with some low-fat soft white cheese, a pinch of cayenne pepper and a squeeze of lemon juice. Blend until smooth, season to taste, and chill.

Meal suggestions

▶ Grilled (allow 3 sardines, 1–2 fillets, or 1 small whole fish per person) served on a bed of crushed hot chick-peas, garlic, and a dash of olive oil with a large mixed salad (for lunch, add some new potatoes)

▶ Soused mackerel with a beetroot, white cabbage, and red onion salad (for lunch, add some plain boiled potatoes)

▶ Fresh or smoked mackerel salad with hard-boiled eggs, spring onions, watercress, tomatoes, and radishes, and a yoghurt dressing flavoured with grated or creamed horseradish (for lunch, add some wholegrain bread)

▶ Smear fish fillets with harissa paste. Sauté in just a little olive oil for about 3 minutes each side until cooked. Serve on a bed of hot haricot, cannellini or borlotti beans with a green bean salad (for lunch, add some couscous).

▶ Grilled or poached kipper with scrambled eggs and a large green salad (for lunch, add some wholemeal toast)

Snack suggestions

▶ A little smoked fish pâté on 2 oatcakes with some slices of cucumber

▶ 1 or 2 canned sardines on fingers of toast

▶ 2 slices cut from a cold soused mackerel on a slice of pumpernickel bread spread with a little low-fat white soft cheese

What to look for
•All fish should look and smell fresh.
•Eyes should be bright, not opaque or sunken.
•Gills should be bright red.
•Skin should be slippery.

Ways to cook or serve
•Grill
•Sauté
•Bake
•Souse
•Salad
•Pâté

Simple ways to flavour
•Herbs (chopped, fresh): dill, tarragon, and parsley as part of a salsa dressing or as a gremolata (with grated lemon zest and some chopped hard-boiled egg), sprinkled over the fish after grilling
•Horseradish and lemon wedges with smoked or plain grilled mackerel or herring
•Spices: harissa paste and spice rubs (a mixture of your chosen spices, or buy a pot of Cajun or jerk spices) rubbed over the fish before grilling or sautéing
•Fresh lemon or lime wedges to squeeze over plain grilled fish

Mackerel with salsa verde

This recipe uses mackerel, but you can use herring fillets in the same way, or try whole sardines and serve with the salsa verde and green beans. Salsa verde is good with all fish, grilled steaks, and even spooned over oysters just before serving.

Makes 4 portions

For the salsa verde:
1 bunch fresh parsley (about 30g)
8 stoned green olives
1 tbsp pickled capers
120ml olive oil
Juice of 1 lemon
2 tbsp white balsamic
Freshly ground black pepper

For the fish:
4 mackerel, each about 250g, cleaned
   and filleted into two fillets
   (or 8 mackerel fillets)
1 tbsp olive oil
Lemon wedges and sprigs of parsley
   to garnish

To serve: green beans and courgettes

1. Put the parsley in a food processor with the olives, capers, oil, lemon juice, and balsamic condiment. Blend until chopped and mixed, stopping the processor if necessary to scrape down the sides. Season with black pepper.
2. Preheat the grill. Rinse the fish and pat dry with kitchen paper. Brush the flesh surfaces with the olive oil.
3. Line the grill with foil. Place the fish, skin-side up, on the grill rack. Grill for 5–6 minutes until the skin is crispy and golden and cooked through. Do not turn the fish over.
4. Transfer to warm plates and spoon the salsa verde around the fish. Garnish with lemon wedges and sprigs of parsley. Serve with the green beans and courgettes.

Lunch only
Cover the mackerel in an oat and seed topping before grilling.

For the coating:
8 tbsp fine oatmeal
2 tbsp sesame seeds
2 tbsp celery seeds

Finely grated zest of 1 lemon
A pinch of salt (optional)
2 tbsp sesame oil

Mix the oatmeal with the seeds, lemon zest, salt if using, and some black pepper. Stir in the sesame oil until well combined. Press the oatmeal mixture all over the flesh (not the skin side) to cover the tops completely. Then cook as instructed in step 4, but with the coated sides up (and the skin sides down on the foil). Serve with new potatoes.

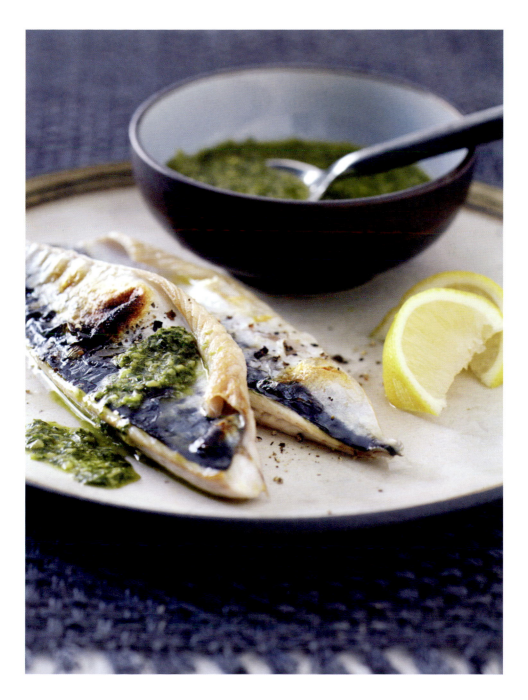

Salmon and trout

These fish vary in their quality and levels of fat (colour isn't an indication of quality with salmon: some wild salmon has a bright, orangey red colour, while other species are pale pink). And although farmed fish has more fat than its wild counterparts, this fat may not be so high in the valuable omega-3 fatty acids that we usually associate with oily fish. This is because some farmed fish are fed on a diet that is plant-based. Wild salmon eat fish, not plants, so their fat content is almost exclusively made of omega-3 fatty acids. If you buy farmed salmon, choose organically farmed fish if possible because it will have been fed on sustainable fish so will have good levels of omega 3.

All fresh salmon and trout are excellent sources of protein, as are smoked salmon and trout – both hot- (cooked) and cold- (raw) smoked – and canned salmon.

Three simple cooking techniques

Poach (for fillets, steaks, or whole fish) Weigh large fish first. Place in a pan or fish kettle and cover with water, fish, or vegetable stock. Place whole fish on kitchen foil that covers the sides of the pan (so you can lift out the cooked fish). Add an onion, 6 peppercorns, and a bay leaf. Bring slowly to the boil, cover, and simmer gently for 3–4 minutes for steaks, fillets, or small fish. Cook large fish for 4 minutes per 450g. Turn off the heat and leave to stand for 10 minutes. Lift out and serve hot, or leave to cool in the liquid, remove, and chill.

Pan-roast (for thick salmon, sea trout steaks, and small whole trout) Preheat the oven to 200°C (Gas 6). Season the steaks. Heat a little olive oil in an ovenproof frying pan. Brown the fish, skin-side down, for 2 minutes only (or on one side if a whole fish). Turn the fish over. Place the pan in the hot oven for 4 minutes or until just cooked. Transfer to plates and pour the juices over.

Bake, stuffed Sauté some finely shredded leek, celery, and carrot in a little olive oil. Add fresh chopped herbs and seasoning. Put small whole fish or cutlets in an oiled roasting tin. Fill the cavities with the stuffing. Pour some stock and apple juice around. Cover the tin with foil and bake at 180°C (Gas 4) for 30 minutes. Remove the foil (or bake in foil parcels) and bake for 10 minutes until lightly golden. Transfer to warm plates. Boil the juices to reduce. Add some half-fat crème fraîche to the juices, if you like. Don't re-boil.

Meal suggestions

▸ Grilled steak or fillet on wilted spinach with quick hollandaise sauce (right) and some grilled tomatoes (for lunch, add some new potatoes)

▸ Poached salmon or trout salad. Poach the fish (left), place while still warm, or cold, on a bed of mixed salad and serve with mayonnaise (for lunch, add some warm new potatoes).

▸ Baked stuffed salmon cutlets (left) with green beans (for lunch, add jacket potatoes)

▸ Smoked salmon and broccoli scrambled eggs. Start scrambling some eggs and when creamy, but only half set, stir in cooked broccoli and smoked salmon trimmings. Cook until just set, but don't overcook. Season well with black pepper (for lunch, add some wholemeal toast).

▸ Pan-roasted steaks or whole small trout with caper dressing. Pan-roast the fish (left), but add some chopped tomatoes, capers, and a little more olive oil before baking. Dust with a few dried chilli flakes and serve with a large green salad with some toasted pumpkin seeds (for lunch, add some couscous).

Snack suggestions

▸ Half a bagel, spread with some low-fat white soft cheese, a lettuce leaf, a few smoked salmon trimmings, a squeeze of lemon juice, and some freshly ground black pepper

▸ Open sandwich of a little canned salmon on rye bread, topped with some sliced cucumber and a squeeze of lemon juice

▸ A little cooked fresh or smoked salmon or trout, flaked, beaten into a little natural yoghurt and some snipped chives and served with some crudités

What to look for
• Fillets, whole fish, salmon steaks or cutlets cut from a section through the fish with a central T-shaped bone, hot-smoked salmon steaks, fillets of smoked trout, raw sliced smoked salmon or whole sides
• If buying whole, the eyes should be bright, not sunken, the gills should be red, and the skin slippery.
• Smoked salmon trimmings are offcuts from sliced sides of salmon. They are inexpensive and fine for omelette fillings, with scrambled eggs, pasta, rice, sandwiches, or pâté.

Ways to cook or serve
• Poach
• Grill
• Bake
• Stir-fry or sauté
• Pan-roast
• Salads
• Pâté (see mackerel, p.98)
• Soup

Simple ways to flavour
• Melted butter or olive oil and toasted almonds
• Capers, chopped fresh tomatoes, and herbs
• Quick hollandaise sauce: whisk 2 eggs in a saucepan with a good squeeze of lemon juice. Gradually whisk in 115g melted butter. Whisk over a very gentle heat until thickened. Do not boil. Season and sharpen with more lemon juice.

Salmon with baby spinach and pumpkin seed pennes

You can also use trout fillets with a few toasted flaked almonds as a change from pumpkin seeds. You can also, if you wish, pile the fish and spinach mixture onto griddled aubergine slices (pp.158–59) before serving for dinner, and omit the penne.

Makes 4 portions

250g wholewheat penne pasta
2 tbsp olive oil
350g salmon fillets, skinned and cut into bite-sized chunks
1 small fresh red chilli, deseeded and chopped
1 garlic clove, finely chopped
250g baby spinach leaves
150ml fish or chicken stock
115g cherry tomatoes, halved

30g stoned sliced or whole stoned black or green olives
1 tbsp pickled capers
A good squeeze of lemon juice
Freshly ground black pepper
3 tbsp pumpkin seeds
2 tbsp toasted pumpkin seed or sesame oil (optional)
Lemon wedges and a few torn fresh basil leaves to garnish

1. Cook the pasta in boiling water, according to the packet directions. Drain.
2. Heat the oil in a large frying pan or wok. Add the salmon, chilli, and garlic and fry, stirring gently, for 1 minute.
3. Add the spinach and stock and simmer, turning over gently for about 2 minutes until beginning to wilt. Gently fold in the pasta and the remaining ingredients except the pumpkin or sesame oil, if using. Toss gently and simmer for 3 minutes until most of the liquid has been absorbed. Pile on warm plates and drizzle with the seed oil, if using. Garnish with lemon wedges and a few torn basil leaves.

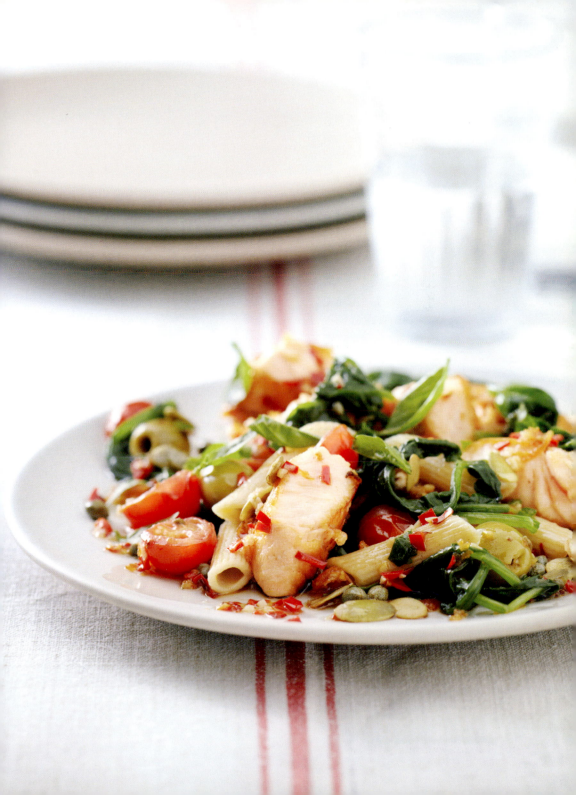

Tuna and swordfish

Fish such as these are meaty and don't fall apart easily like more delicate species, so they are ideal served as whole steaks or cut into pieces to add to other ingredients.

Tuna and swordfish both have a strong, sweet taste, so they can take more robust flavours. Always cook these fish lightly or they quickly become dry and unpalatable. Fresh tuna, in particular, should be served while it is still pink in the middle. If you buy canned tuna, choose fish in water or olive oil rather than brine (to reduce the salt content) and drain well before use.

Unlike other oily fish, tuna and swordfish are great sources of omega-3 fatty acids. Responsible fishing is vital, so buy line-caught or farmed tuna; when buying canned tuna, check it is labelled dolphin-friendly and from a sustainable source.

Three simple cooking techniques

Griddle Marinate first, if you like (see panel, opposite, or brush with olive oil and season with freshly ground black pepper. Heat a griddle pan until very hot (when your hand feels hot when you hold it 5cm above the surface). Griddle for 2 minutes on each side – and no more – for tuna steaks so that they are striped brown on the outside, but still slightly pink in the centre. Griddle swordfish steaks for 3 minutes on each side.

Roast Heat a little olive oil in a roasting tin at 200°C (Gas 6). Season the steaks. When the oil is sizzling hot, add the fish, turn it over in the hot oil, and roast in the oven for 15–20 minutes.

Stew Cut the fish into chunks. Simmer vegetables of your choice in a little fish or vegetable stock with a bouquet garni until just tender. Add the fish and cook for a further 3–5 minutes, and no more. Discard the bouquet garni. Add some low-fat crème fraîche if you like. Taste and re-season, then add some chopped fresh parsley.

Meal suggestions

- Tuna carpaccio: prepare as for beef carpaccio (p.46), slice thinly, arrange on a platter with plenty of rocket and baby cherry tomatoes, drizzle with olive oil and lime juice and scatter over fresh Parmesan shavings (for lunch, add a wholemeal baguette).

- Roasted steaks drizzled with balsamic vinegar, and with cherry tomatoes roasted in the same tray, with green beans and celeriac wedges (p.144) (for lunch, add sweet potato wedges)

- Tuna and sweetcorn bake: mix canned tuna with some canned sweetcorn in water, or thawed frozen kernels. Stir in half-fat crème fraîche and some grated Cheddar cheese. Season and top with sliced tomatoes and some extra cheese. Bake at 190°C (Gas 5) until golden. Serve with a green salad (for lunch, stir the mixture through cooked wholewheat spaghetti or pasta shapes before topping and baking).

- Salade Niçoise: use stir-fried fresh chunks or canned tuna. Mix torn salad leaves with sliced red onion, black olives, tomatoes, and cucumber. Add the fish and some anchovy fillets, if you like. Toss with French dressing. Top with quartered hard-boiled eggs (for lunch, add warm or cold new potatoes to the salad).

- Peasant-style sautéed steaks: fry steaks in a little olive oil for 2–3 minutes on each side until golden. Transfer to warm plates. Add some chopped garlic, fresh parsley, a little more olive oil, and lemon juice to the pan juices. Season, heat through, and spoon over. Serve with a large mixed salad (for lunch, add some wholegrain bread).

Snack suggestions

- Tuna dip: blend canned tuna with some natural yoghurt and a dash of tomato purée and Worcestershire sauce. Store in the fridge to use over a few days. Serve a spoonful with crudités or on crackers.

- Mix a little canned tuna with some drained canned sweetcorn in water, or thawed frozen kernels. Moisten with mayonnaise and spoon onto wholegrain crackers.

- Blend a can of tuna and a can of white beans to a paté. Season and flavour with garlic, lemon juice, and a splash of olive oil. Store in the fridge and spread on celery sticks.

What to look for
- Fresh tuna and swordfish steaks should have very little smell and should look moist. Tuna should be a good red colour; swordfish should be pale pink with dark streaks.
- Avoid if the steaks are drying out. If buying frozen, it is best to thaw before use.

Ways to cook or serve
- Salad
- Grill
- Griddle
- Stir-fry or sauté
- Roast
- Stew or casserole

Simple ways to flavour
- Simple marinade: olive oil, garlic, lemon or lime juice, and some dried chilli flakes
- Tandoori paste with natural yoghurt and chopped fresh coriander as a marinade before grilling or roasting
- Olives, tomatoes, capers, and onions with canned or fresh tuna
- Cheese and sweetcorn with canned tuna

Seared sweet-and-sour tuna steaks

These are equally delicious made with swordfish steaks (or you could use chicken breasts, beaten flat, or Quorn steaks. Quorn takes the same time to cook, but the others need to be cooked through – about 3 minutes on each side).

Makes 4 portions

4 tbsp balsamic vinegar
4 tbsp sunflower oil
4 tbsp soy sauce, plus extra
  for sprinkling
1 tbsp tomato purée
1 large garlic clove, crushed
2.5cm piece fresh root ginger, grated

4 fresh tuna steaks
1 large carrot
1 large courgette
2 tbsp snipped fresh chives
4 large handfuls of fresh bean sprouts
2 tbsp pickled ginger slivers
A few whole chive stalks to garnish

1. Mix the vinegar, oil, soy sauce, tomato purée, garlic, and fresh ginger together in a large shallow container with a lid.
2. Add the tuna steaks, turning them over to coat them in the marinade. Then cover and leave to marinate in the fridge for 1–2 hours.
3. Pare the carrot and courgette into thin ribbons with a potato peeler. Blanch the carrot and courgette ribbons in a pan of boiling water for 2 minutes. Drain and return to the pan. Add the chives, bean sprouts, and half the ginger slivers (chopped if necessary) and toss with a sprinkling of soy sauce.
4. Heat a non-stick griddle pan. Drain the tuna, reserving the marinade in the container, and sear for 1 ½ minutes on each side in the hot pan until brown-striped on the outside and still slightly pink in the centre.
5. Pile vegetable ribbons onto warm plates. Top with the tuna. Mix 120ml of water with the remaining marinade in the container, add to the griddle pan, swirl round, then spoon over the tuna. Top with the remaining pickled ginger and lay 2–3 chive stalks across each steak.

Lunch only

Serve with 3 bundles (250g) of soba (buckwheat) noodles, or use udon (brown rice) noodles and use only 1 carrot and 1 courgette. Cook the noodles before griddling the tuna. Add the carrot and courgette ribbons to the noodles 2 minutes before the end of the cooking time, then pile the noodles and vegetable ribbons onto warm plates before topping with the tuna.

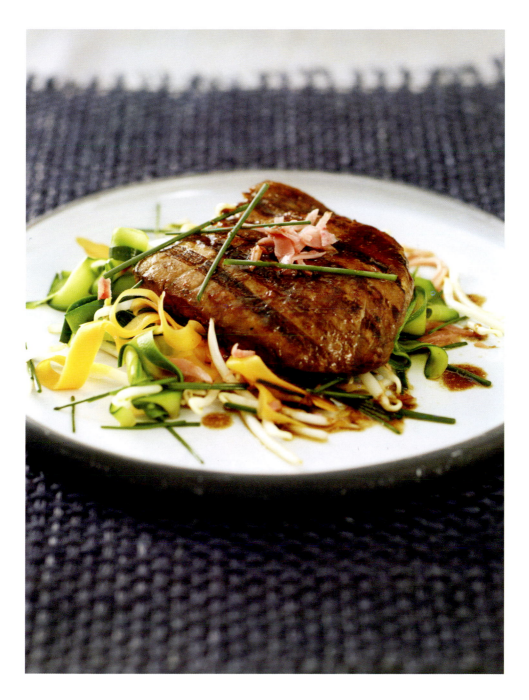

Large white meaty fish fillets

This group incorporates the cod family, which, apart from cod, comprises haddock, pollack, whiting, and coley. Monkfish, halibut, and turbot have also been included in this group, as they can all be cooked in similar ways although they are different species. They vary considerably in price. Coley and pollack are inexpensive, while turbot and monkfish are much dearer but taste delicious. All are worth including in a varied diet.

Smoked fish such as haddock, cod, and whiting are also suitable, but beware of any fillets that have been dyed bright yellow; choose instead naturally smoked, undyed smoked varieties, which have a pale, creamy colour and don't contain chemical additives. These fish are all great sources of protein and, although not as high in omega-3 fatty acids as oily fish, they are still an excellent choice.

Three simple cooking techniques

Braise Sauté some finely diced vegetables of your choice in a little olive oil in a flameproof casserole until almost soft. Top with the fish. Pour some apple juice and/or stock around the fish and vegetables. Add herbs of your choice. Season. Cover and cook in a moderate oven for about 40 minutes, or until the fish is tender and the vegetables are cooked through. Stir in some half-fat crème fraîche if you like.

Thai-style curry Mix some green curry paste with coconut milk in a saucepan. Add some chopped lemon grass and a splash of thai fish sauce. Add some diced fish. Bring to the boil, reduce the heat, and simmer for 5 minutes.

Ceviche Use very fresh fish. Cut the fish in slices, then thin strips. Put in a bowl with a chopped fat green and red fresh chilli, some diced red pepper, and some thinly sliced onion. Drizzle well with fresh lime juice. Toss gently and season. Cover and chill for about 2 hours until the fish is opaque. Drizzle with olive oil and add lots of torn fresh coriander or flat-leaf parsley.

Meal suggestions

▸ Provençal-style stew: make a tomato stew with fresh or canned chopped tomatoes, onions, and garlic. Add cubes of fish and simmer for 5 minutes until just cooked. Add some olives and chopped fresh parsley. Serve with a green salad (for lunch, spoon over brown rice).

▸ Thai green fish curry: make as before (opposite), but add some cooked green beans and broccoli at the last minute (for lunch, spoon over wholewheat noodles).

▸ Ceviche served spooned over a bed of salad leaves (for lunch, add wholegrain bread)

▸ Poached smoked fish on wilted spinach, topped with poached eggs, and served with pan-sautéed cherry tomatoes drizzled with balsamic vinegar (for lunch, add wholemeal toast)

▸ Chunky fish kebabs (use cod loin, monkfish or turbot): marinate the fish in olive oil, chilli, and lime juice. Grill on oiled kitchen foil until golden and cooked through, brushing with any leftover marinade as they cook. Serve with satay sauce on a bed of steamed pak choi (for lunch, add some udon [brown rice] noodles, dressed in sesame oil).

Snack suggestions

▸ A little poached smoked fish, flaked and moistened with mayonnaise, on a large wholegrain cracker

▸ A little leftover ceviche in half a wholemeal pitta bread

▸ Any cold cooked white fish, mixed with some chopped peanuts and a pinch of dried chilli flakes, spooned into a large scooped-out tomato

What to look for
•Firm, white moist flesh
•No strong odour
•Avoid if discoloured or drying out.
•Frozen fish is fine, but fresh is best; eat it on the day you buy.
•Coley looks a bit grey when raw, but cooks white and has a good texture and flavour.

Ways to cook or serve
•Steam
•Poach
•Sauté
•Pan-roast
•Bake or roast
•Stew, casserole, or braise
•Curry
•Ceviche
•Kebabs

Simple ways to flavour
•Chopped tomatoes, onions, garlic, peppers, and olives cooked as a stew
•Added to a vegetable curry
•Raw cured ham (trimmed of fat) wrapped around the fish and topped with melting cheese before grilling or roasting

Hearty fish and baby vegetable stew

Use any chunky white fish or a mixture of white fish and salmon for this dish. The important thing to ensure is that the vegetables are tender before you add the fish for the last few minutes so it doesn't overcook.

Makes 4 portions

1 tbsp olive oil
1 onion, chopped
2 beefsteak tomatoes, skinned
    and chopped
4 canned anchovy fillets, chopped
    or 2 tsp anchovy essence or paste
12 baby carrots, topped and tailed
6 baby turnips, peeled and halved
115g baby corn ears, halved
55g French beans, cut in short lengths

115g button mushrooms
600ml fish or vegetable stock
2 tbsp tomato purée
1 bay leaf
Freshly ground black pepper
450g meaty white fish fillet, cut into
    bite-sized chunks
200g raw king prawns
A little chopped fresh parsley
    to garnish

1. Heat the oil in a large saucepan and fry the onion gently for 2 minutes, stirring until softened, but not browned.
2. Add the tomatoes and cook, stirring for 1 minute.
3. Add the remaining ingredients except the fish and prawns. Bring to the boil, reduce the heat, cover, and simmer gently for 20–30 minutes until the vegetables are tender.
4. Add the fish and prawns and continue to cook for 5 minutes until they are just cooked through. Discard the bay leaf. Taste and re-season if necessary.
5. Ladle into warm bowls and sprinkle with the chopped parsley.

Lunch only
Serve with wholegrain bread.

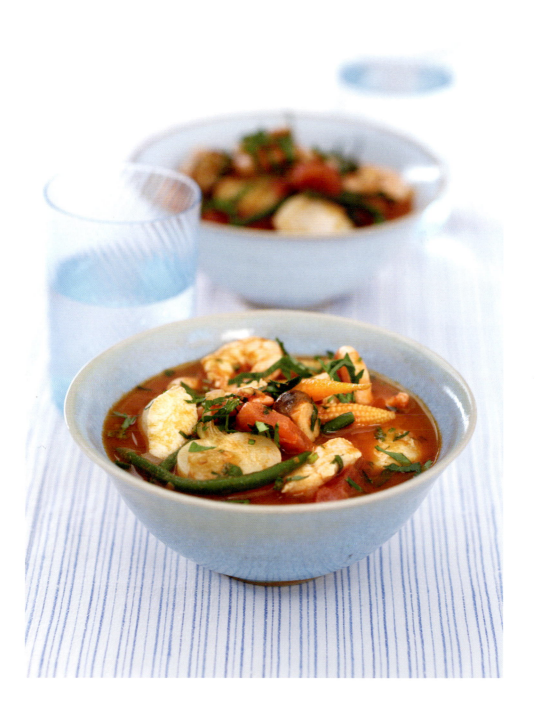

Small whole white fish

This group covers all the delicious fish that, while still fairly small, can be cooked and eaten whole, but are also sold as fillets from larger fish. These fish include sea bass, all the breams, red snapper, red and grey mullet, red gurnard, and John Dory. They all have excellent eating quality, although red gurnard tends to have quite a few bones, so it is most popular eaten in classic fish stews along with other species.

Many fishmongers will clean and scale (when necessary) the fish for you, but it is quite straightforward if you need to do it yourself: to clean the fish, make a slit along the belly and pull out the guts. Then rinse under cold water and dry with kitchen paper. To remove large scales, simply place the fish on some newspaper, hold it at the tail end (dip your fingers in salt first to stop them sliding), and scrape the fish from tail to head end with a knife. Rinse and pat dry with kitchen paper (for oily fish, see p.98).

Three simple cooking techniques

Bake whole, stuffed Trim the fins and any spines from the fish. Gently open the fish up and fill with your chosen stuffing. Season, wrap in oiled kitchen foil, and bake at 180°C (Gas 4) for about 20 minutes.

Sauté fillets Season and flavour as desired (opposite). Heat a little olive or sunflower oil in a frying pan. Fry the fillets, skin-side down first, until crisp and golden underneath, then flip over with a fish slice and quickly cook on the other side.

Steam Fill whole fish with fresh herbs, or season fillets with spices or chopped herbs of your choosing. Place the fish side by side on some oiled greaseproof paper in a steamer, in an electric steamer, or in a metal colander over a pan of simmering water. Cover and steam for 5–15 minutes, depending on the thickness of the fish, until cooked through.

Meal suggestions

▸ Grilled fillets on a bed of crushed celeriac with a natural yoghurt and chopped fresh dill dressing. Serve with green beans and carrots (for lunch, cook potatoes with the celeriac mash and crush them together).

▸ Steamed whole fish stuffed with sautéed celery, carrot, and spring onion strips, and flavoured with grated ginger. Sprinkle with soy sauce before steaming. Serve on a bed of carrot and courgette ribbons (for lunch, add soba [buckwheat] noodles, dressed with soy sauce and lime juice).

▸ Sautéed fillets, rubbed with harissa paste before sautéeing. Serve on steamed mixed diced vegetables and garnish with lime wedges (for lunch, serve with couscous).

▸ Baked whole fish, stuffed first with chopped mushrooms, moistened with crème fraîche and flavoured with chopped fresh tarragon, served on wilted spinach (for lunch, add some new potatoes)

▸ Fillets braised on a bed of chopped canned tomatoes, olives, peppers, and onions (moistened with a little apple juice only), and flavoured with a little chopped rosemary. Serve with a green salad (for lunch, add some brown rice).

Snack suggestions

▸ Half a cold cooked fillet, flaked on tapenade (olive paste) spread on a large wholegrain cracker

▸ A little leftover braised fish with tomatoes (above), flaked and mixed with a little cold cooked brown rice

▸ A little cold cooked fish, mixed with mayonnaise and a little tomato purée, with some chopped cornichons and some shredded lettuce in half a wholewheat pitta bread

What to look for
•Choose whole fish with bright, prominent eyes and red gills.
•The fish should smell of the ocean, but not 'fishy'.

Ways to cook or serve
•Steam
•Braise
•Grill
•Sauté
•Bake

Simple ways to flavour
•A mixture of some shredded or finely diced softened carrot, celery, parsnip, turnip, celeriac, and onion or spring onion for stuffing or braising
•Herbs (chopped fresh): dill, tarragon, parsley, and thyme
•Spices: a mixture of smoked and sweet paprika with some salt and pepper, or harissa paste, as a rub before grilling

Whole fish parcels with fragrant herbs, courgettes, and lemon

This is a lovely way to cook any small whole fish, but you can use fillets if you prefer. The pleasure comes in opening the foil parcels at the table and inhaling all the fragrant steam that rises from the cooked fish.

Makes 4 portions

2 tbsp olive oil
2 courgettes, thinly sliced
4 whole round fish, such as sea bream, sea bass, red mullet (each about 350g), cleaned and scaled
1 x 50g can anchovy fillets, drained

2 tbsp chopped fresh tarragon
2 tbsp chopped fresh parsley
2 tbsp chopped fresh thyme
1 small lemon, sliced
Freshly ground black pepper
4 tbsp apple juice

To serve: a green salad

1. Preheat the oven to 220°C (Gas 7). Cut 4 large pieces of kitchen foil about 30 x 40cm in size. Brush the foil with olive oil. Lay the courgettes in a single layer, slightly overlapping, in the centre of each piece of foil as a base for the fish. Leave plenty of foil free round the edges.
2. Wash the fish inside and out and pat dry with kitchen paper.
3. Lay the fish on the courgettes. Lay the anchovies over the fish, then add the herbs and then the lemon slices. Add a good grinding of black pepper and spoon a tablespoon of apple juice and a tablespoon of water over each piece of fish. Draw the foil up over the fish and fold and scrunch up the edges to seal the parcel all the way along. Fold and scrunch the ends, too, then place on a baking sheet.
4. Bake in the oven for 30 minutes. Transfer the parcels to plates and open at the table. Serve with a green salad.

Lunch only
Serve with new potatoes.

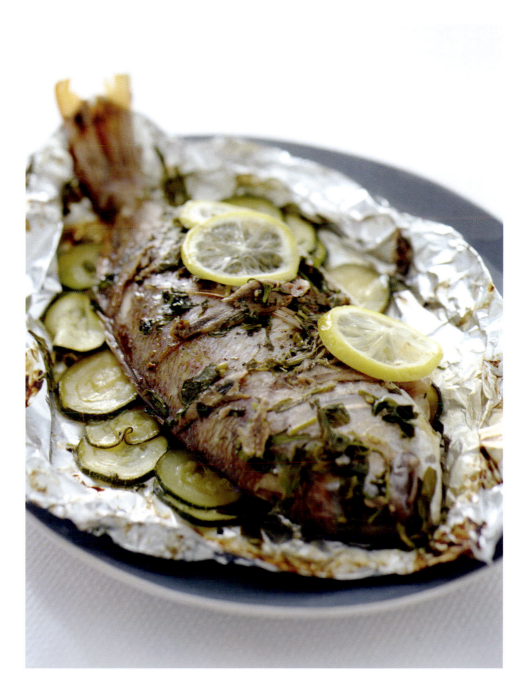

Delicate flat fish

This group includes Dover sole, but also more inexpensive cousins such as lemon sole, plaice, dab, brill, and flounder. These flat fish all have a soft, delicate flesh and a sweet, mild flavour. They are all interchangeable for cooking and are available as fillets or as whole fish. If they have not been prepared by the fishmonger to cook whole, cut off the fins all round with scissors, but leave the head intact.

To skin the fish at home, put the fillets on a board or the kitchen work surface, skin-side down. Make a nick at the tail end. Dip your fingers in salt (so they won't slip) before holding the skin at the tail end, then, holding the skin all the while, ease a knife between the skin and the flesh all the way along the length of the fish. If buying fillets, the white skin on the fillets from the underside of the fish doesn't need removing before cooking, but most people prefer to remove the dark, tough upper skin, as it is rather more unpalatable and doesn't look attractive.

Three simple cooking techniques

Steam Season fillets and roll up skinned side in (or white skin side in). Place on a lightly oiled dinner plate. Add a splash of milk. Cover with a lid or another dinner plate and steam over a pan of simmering water for about 15 minutes until cooked through. Alternatively, prepare as above and put in an electric steamer. Use the cooking milk to make a sauce, if you like.

Grill (whole) Trim the fish and brush with a little melted butter or olive or sunflower oil. Season. Place on kitchen foil on the grill rack and grill for 5–6 minutes each side until cooked through and lightly golden. Do not overcook.

Bake If serving for lunch, coat fillets in beaten egg and a crumb or a cooked couscous crust. If not, simply season. Heat a little sunflower or olive oil and butter in a roasting tin in the oven at 190°C (Gas 5). Put the fish in the tin and roast for 10–15 minutes (depending on size), carefully turning over once (cook small whole fish in the same way).

Meal suggestions

▶ Grilled whole flat fish brushed with melted butter, sprinkled with fresh parsley, and served with steamed carrots and mangetout (for lunch, add some new potatoes)

▶ Steamed rolls in a sauce of mayonnaise thinned with the cooking milk and a little half-fat crème fraîche and chopped cucumber, flavoured with chopped fresh or dried dill, heated through and spooned over. Serve with peas and courgettes (for lunch, add some potato and sweet potato mash mixed together and flavoured with chives).

▶ Whole baked fish (opposite) with prawn sauce (right). Serve with roasted asparagus and cherry tomatoes (for lunch, add some saffron-flavoured brown rice).

▶ Steamed rolls with tomato mayonnaise and toasted almonds: cook the fillet rolls and allow to cool in their liquid. Thin the mayonnaise with the cooled cooking milk and flavour with tomato purée and Worcestershire sauce. Put the fish rolls on a bed of mixed salad. Spoon the sauce over and top with toasted flaked almonds (for lunch, add some wholemeal bread).

▶ Baked fillets (opposite) with tartare sauce, celeriac chips (p.144) and peas (for lunch, substitute baked potato wedges [p.144] for the celeriac chips)

Snack suggestions

▶ An open sandwich of a little cooked flat fish in tartare sauce (right) spread on half a slice of wholemeal bread

▶ A little cooked flat fish mixed with some mashed cooked peas and chopped mint and rolled up in a lettuce leaves

▶ A little cooked flat fish mixed with mayonnaise and a splash of Tabasco in half a wholemeal pitta with some shredded lettuce

What to look for
•Choose fish that feel firm and moist, but not slimy, and with a sweet, fresh smell.

Ways to cook or serve
•Grill
•Sauté
•Bake
•Poach (fillets)
•Steam (fillets)
•Cooked and served cold as a salad

Simple ways to flavour
•Melted butter and chopped parsley with a squeeze of lemon juice
•A quick sauce of prawns tossed in half-fat crème fraîche thinned with milk and flavoured with anchovy essence, some snipped chives, and dill, heated gently in a saucepan
•Tartare sauce (chopped capers, cornichons, and parsley mixed into mayonnaise and thinned with a little of the vinegar from the jar of capers)

Grilled plaice with egg, lemon, and watercress sauce

This recipe is good with any flat fish. If you aren't fond of watercress, use chopped fresh parsley instead. If you are hungry, make some celeriac mash to serve with it.

Makes 4 portions

1 egg
4 good handfuls watercress (about 30g)
Finely grated zest and juice of
    ½ lemon
200ml half-fat crème fraîche
4 tbsp milk

Freshly ground black pepper
4 small plaice on the bone
    (about 350g each)
1–2 tbsp sunflower oil
Extra sprigs of watercress to garnish

To serve: baby corn cobs and carrots

1. Boil the egg in water for 5 minutes, then drain and place in cold water. Shell and finely chop.
2. Finely chop the watercress, discarding any thick stalks. Mix with the egg, lemon zest and juice, crème fraîche, and milk in a saucepan and season with black pepper. Do not heat yet.
3. Preheat the grill. Trim the fins off the plaice with scissors, if not already done. Line the grill with foil and lay the fish on the rack, dark skin-side up first. Brush all over with oil and season with black pepper. Grill the fish for 5–6 minutes each side until golden and just cooked through.
4. When the fish is nearly cooked, heat the sauce, stirring gently, but do not boil. Transfer the fish to warm plates and spoon the sauce over. Garnish with extra sprigs of watercress and serve.

Lunch only
Serve with mashed potatoes.
Make the mash by boiling 3–4 large potatoes or 1 large celeriac, peeled and cut in small chunks. When cooked until tender, mash with a small knob of butter and plenty of freshly ground black pepper.

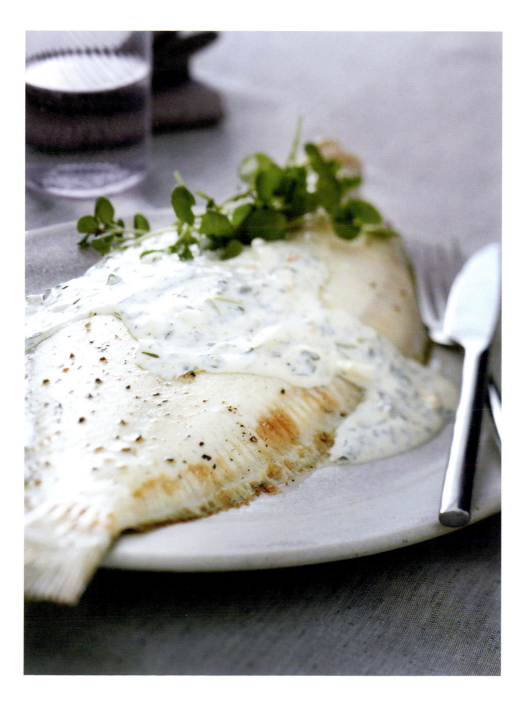

Seafood: molluscs

This group includes bivalves such as mussels, oysters, and gastropods – the snail-like creatures such as winkles and whelks – and cephalopods such as squid and cuttlefish. They are all delicious to eat, quick to cook, and are highly nutritious.

Some molluscs are still gathered from the wild, but Pacific oysters and mussels are now extensively farmed and available all year round (although there are a few wild beds still around producing fabulous native oysters and wild mussels). Several varieties of clams and razor clams are available, and they are also sold canned and as clam juice, with or without tomato. Large king scallops and smaller queen scallops are farmed all year and also available frozen. Whelks, winkles, and cockles are available in season, and cockles are also available in jars. Baby and larger squid are available fresh and frozen, and also sold in rings.

Three simple cooking techniques

Boil (whelks and winkles) Put a halved onion, a few peppercorns, and a bouquet garni in a saucepan of water. Bring to the boil, add the shellfish, and boil for 5 minutes for winkles, 8 minutes for whelks. Drain and discard the flavourings. Serve warm or cold. Pick off the sucker and pull out the meat with a pin or picker.

Steam (bivalves) Soften a chopped onion, shallot, or other flavourings such as chopped garlic, carrot, celery, or fennel in a little olive oil or butter and oil. Add about 1 cm of liquid – such as water, stock, or apple juice – and some black pepper. Add the shellfish, bring to the boil, cover, and steam, shaking the pan occasionally, for 5 minutes until they open. Discard any that stay closed.

Shuck (oysters, scallops) With your hand protected by an oven glove or cloth, hold the oyster or scallop firmly, flat side up. Push the point of a sharp knife between the shells, close to the hinge. Twist upwards, pushing towards the hinge until it breaks. Lift off the top shell (taking care not to spill the oyster juices). Loosen the meat from the shell with the knife. For scallops, peel off the covering membrane and remove the black intestine. Oysters can be served raw, but scallops must be cooked first.

Meal suggestions

▶ Clam or mussel chowder: diced onion, carrot, and celeriac softened in butter or sunflower oil and simmered in fish stock with some dried oregano, a bay leaf, and seasoning until tender. Add some canned clams, diced lean raw cured ham, and half-fat crème fraîche and heat through (for lunch, add some wholegrain bread).

▶ Scallops or squid sautéed very quickly in olive oil with spring onions, dried chilli flakes, and a squeeze of lime juice served with a large green salad including avocado (for lunch, add some saffron rice)

▶ Mussel salad: steam some mussels, remove from their shells, and mix with diced peppers, cucumber, chopped spring onion, peas, and quinoa cooked in stock with some saffron and allowed to cool.

▶ Queen scallops poached briefly in milk with mushrooms and flavoured with a bay leaf, covered with a half-fat crème fraîche and cheese sauce thinned with the cooking milk. Top with grated Parmesan cheese and bake until golden. Serve with a large salad (for lunch, add new potatoes).

▶ Pasta with clams or cockles (lunch only): steam the shellfish in onion-flavoured stock and drain, reserving the stock. Cook the pasta in the reserved liquid with diced carrot and celery. Mix the cockles or clams into the pasta and sprinkle with plenty of chopped fresh parsley and dill.

Snack suggestions

▶ A small dish of cockles in vinegar, seasoned with freshly ground black pepper with 2 rice cakes

▶ A dish of whelks or winkles drizzled with a little garlic oil and a small slice of wholemeal bread

▶ A glass of clam and tomato juice with a few drops of Tabasco sauce and a stick of celery

What to look for
•All molluscs should smell very fresh and of the sea. Avoid any that are very open or damaged. If they don't close when tapped, they are already dead. Serve each oyster in the round-sided part of the oyster shell so it remains surrounded by its juice. Eat on the day you buy them.

Ways to cook or serve
•Steam
•Boil
•Salad
•Sauté
•Raw (oysters)
•Grill (oysters)
•Griddle (squid)

Simple ways to flavour
•Olive oil, garlic, chopped fresh parsley, and lemon with squid, mussels, clams, or scallops
•Lime juice, chilli, and olive oil with squid, mussels, clams or scallops
•Finely chopped shallots, wine vinegar, and freshly ground black pepper with raw oysters, cooked whelks, winkles, or cockles
•Top oysters with a few drops of Tabasco, a little half-fat crème fraîche, and some Parmesan (or other Italian hard cheese) and grill just until sizzling

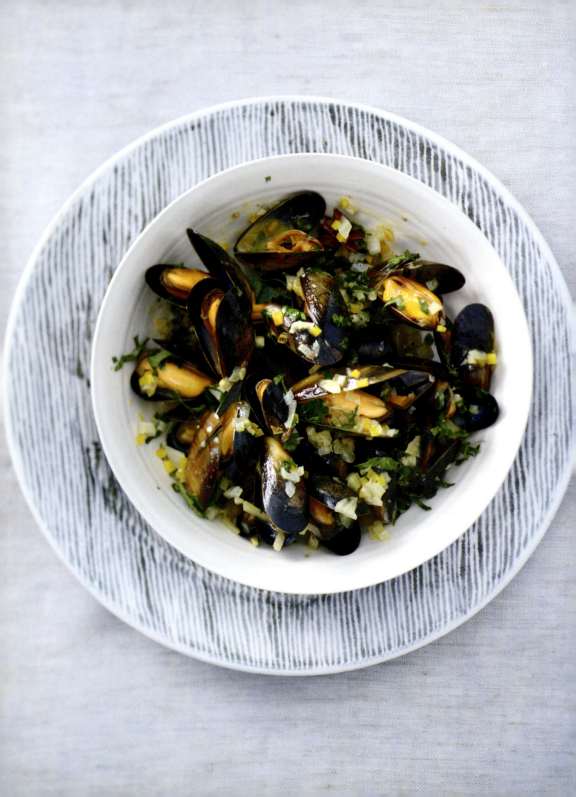

Steamed mussels with fennel and star anise

You can use clams or even cockles for this dish instead of mussels, if you prefer. Serve with a green salad that includes some ripe avocado.

Makes 4 portions

1.8kg fresh mussels in their shells
1 tbsp olive oil
2 shallots, finely chopped
1 garlic clove, finely chopped
1 carrot, finely chopped
1 head of fennel (with the green fronds trimmed and reserved), finely chopped

2 star anise
150ml pure apple juice
Juice of ½ lemon
Freshly ground black pepper
A handful chopped fresh parsley

To serve: a green salad with avocado

1. If you have time, put the mussels in a large bowl, cover with cold water and sprinkle with oatmeal or rolled oats (which helps to clean them). Leave for an hour or more.
2. Scrub the mussels and pull off the 'beard' attached to each shell. Discard any that are broken or open and won't close when tapped sharply with a knife.
3. Heat the oil in a large saucepan. Add the shallots, garlic, carrot, and fennel and cook very gently in the covered pan for 5 minutes to soften (but do not allow the ingredients to brown).
4. Add the star anise, mussels, apple juice, lemon juice, 150ml of water, and some freshly ground black pepper. Bring to the boil, cover, and cook for 5 minutes, shaking the pan occasionally.
5. Ladle the mussels into large bowls, adding all the juices. Discard the star anise and any mussels that remain closed. Sprinkle with the chopped fresh parsley and chopped reserved green fennel fronds and serve straight away.

Lunch only
Serve with wholemeal baguette or spiced wedges (p.144).

Seafood: crustaceans

This group of seafood with hard outer shells is mostly caught fresh in North Atlantic waters (although large tiger prawns are from warmer waters). Prawns are high in cholesterol, but this should not affect your blood cholesterol levels.

Brown crabs are fat, squat, and meaty. They are usually sold cooked and can be bought 'dressed'. Spider crab, a sweet white meat that is usually bought cooked, is more fiddly to eat. Lobster is a succulent, rich meat. Cook it yourself, or buy ready-cooked. Langoustine is a tiny relative of the lobster, also known as scampi. There is a lot of body to tail so you don't get much for your money, but they are delicious. They are the same colour raw as cooked. North Atlantic prawns are small, while tiger prawns are much bigger. They are both available raw and ready-cooked. Brown shrimps are fiddly to peel, but have an excellent flavour. Freshwater crayfish look like little lobsters. The tails are also sold ready-cooked.

Three simple cooking techniques

Boil It is considered humane to comatose lobsters, crabs, langoustine, or freshwater crayfish first: put lobsters or crabs in the freezer for 2 hours, and crayfish or langoustines for 45 minutes, until they are almost frozen. Then plunge into boiling salted water in a covered pan. Boil for just a minute or two for prawns or shrimps, 2–3 minutes for langoustines, 5 minutes for crayfish, and 10 minutes per 500g for lobster or crab.

Sauté Heat a little olive oil or butter and oil in a frying pan. Add cooked or raw crustaceans and seasoning of your choice. Sauté quickly for 1–2 minutes, tossing and stirring until hot if already cooked or pink, if cooking from raw.

To dress a cooked crab Twist off the two large claws. Pull off the legs. Pull the body away from the top shell. Remove the intestines stuck in the shell or clinging to the body. Scrape off any dark meat, then discard the intestines. Scoop out the dark meat from the shell. Discard the gills (dead men's fingers) from the body. Crack the claws and legs and remove meat. Pick out bits of white meat from the body. Mix the dark meat with a few wholemeal breadcrumbs and chopped parsley. Season well. Add a pinch of cayenne. Wash the shell. Spoon the dark meat into the centre and the white meat either side.

Meal suggestions

▶ Crustacean salad: simply cooked crustaceans on a bed of lettuce with tomatoes, cucumber, radishes, chopped spring onion, and mayonnaise or French dressing (for lunch, add some wholemeal bread with a scraping of butter)

▶ Avocado salad: slice a whole avocado with any crustaceans tossed in Marie Rose sauce (p.183) with plenty of salad leaves tossed in a little lemon juice and black pepper and some cherry tomatoes (for lunch, add some wholegrain bread).

▶ Prawn and barley pilaf (for lunch only): simmer barley in coconut milk with a dash of turmeric, chilli powder, cumin, and some chopped spring onions. Add some raw king prawns for the last few minutes of cooking. Serve with a green salad.

▶ Seafood pasta (for lunch only): simmer wholewheat pasta shapes in 2½ times as much fish or chicken stock in a covered pan with a pinch of saffron, chopped spring onion, diced peppers, and some peas. When the pasta is cooked and the stock nearly absorbed, stir in some cooked seafood and leave to stand for 5 minutes (also good cold).

▶ Seafood stew: simmer a selection of baby vegetables in stock with a bay leaf until tender. Throw in some crustaceans and some diced white fish or salmon. Simmer for a few minutes longer. Discard the bay leaf. Serve topped with a spoonful of garlic-flavoured mayonnaise (for lunch, add some baby potatoes or serve with some rye bread).

Snack suggestions

▶ A little white crabmeat or a few chopped prawns or shrimps mixed with some low-fat soft cheese and spread on 2 oatcakes

▶ An open sandwich of a few prawns or crab mixed with mayonnaise and some sliced cucumber

▶ Some chopped prawns or shrimps with some shredded lettuce and a little chilli-flavoured yoghurt in half a wholemeal pitta

What to look for
•All crustaceans should smell very fresh and of the sea. Avoid any that are damaged.

Ways to cook or serve
Must be cooked before eating
•Boil
•Sauté
•Stir-fry
•Grill
•Bake
•Soup
•Stew, casserole, or curry
•Salad
•Sandwiches
•Mousse
•Potted

Simple ways to flavour
•Chilli- and garlic-flavoured olive oil or melted butter over grilled or sautéed crustaceans
•Tartare sauce or mayonnaise (plain or Marie Rose, p.183) with all crustaceans except lobster
•Curry spices, coconut milk, and fresh coriander in curries and pilaf

Sizzled prawns with leeks and omelette ribbons

This recipe is equally delicious if you substitute the prawns with squid rings, langoustine tails, or scallops. If you aren't keen on chilli, try adding some celery seeds to taste instead.

Makes 4 portions

4 eggs
Freshly ground black pepper
2 tsp Thai fish sauce
2 leeks, trimmed
400g raw king prawns

6 tbsp olive oil
115g button mushrooms, sliced
Juice of 1 lime
¼ tsp dried chilli flakes
Lime wedges to garnish

1. Beat one of the eggs in a small bowl with a splash of water. Season with black pepper and few drops of Thai fish sauce. Heat about 1 tsp olive oil in an omelette pan. Add the egg mixture and fry, lifting and stirring until golden underneath and just set. Flip over and cook the other side. Slide out of the pan onto a plate. Keep warm while you make three further omelettes in the same way. Roll each omelette up and cut it into thin ribbons. Put back on the plate, cover with kitchen foil, and keep warm while you cook the prawns and leeks.
2. Wash the leeks well, then split in half lengthways then into 4 equal lengths. Cut each length into thin strips.
3. Pat the prawns dry on kitchen paper. Heat half the oil in a wok or large frying pan. Add the leeks and mushrooms and stir-fry for 1 minute. Remove from the pan with a slotted spoon.
4. Add the remaining oil and heat well. Add the prawns and stir-fry for a further 1½ minutes, or until just pink all over and sizzling. Return the leek mixture to the pan and toss gently.
5. Add the remaining fish sauce, the lime juice, chilli flakes, and a good grinding of black pepper. Toss all the ingredients briefly.
6. Pile the omelette ribbons into bowls. Spoon the prawn mixture on top. Garnish each bowl with a lime wedge and serve straight away.

Lunch only

Omit the omelette ribbons and serve with udon (brown rice) noodles instead. Cook three bundles of noodles (250g) in boiling water for 8 minutes. Drain and return to the pan. Add 1 tsp of the fish sauce and toss gently. When the prawns are cooked, spoon the noodles into bowls and top with the prawn mixture.

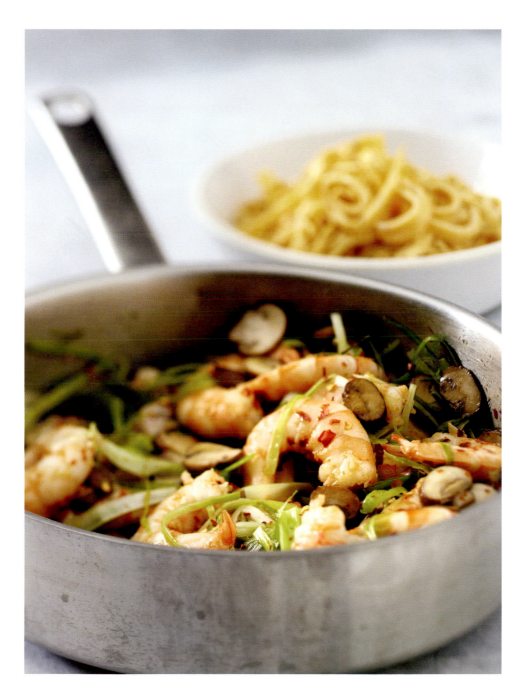

Barley and oats

Barley is often overlooked in favour of couscous and bulgur wheat, but it is a delicious and useful grain that is easy to cook and cheap to buy. We tend to eat oats for breakfast only, but oats are also good for coating and topping foods and for baking.

Both pot barley and pearl barley have a delicious nutty texture and flavour. Pot barley is the whole grain, while pearl barley has had the husks removed. Barley flakes and flour are also available (however, barley is low in protein, so it doesn't make good bread on its own).

The soluble fibre in oats and oat bran have been found to help reduce blood cholesterol levels. Store all these grains in airtight containers in a cool, dark place.

Three simple cooking techniques

Steam (barley) Place 1 part barley to 3 parts water or stock in a pan or stock. Stir, bring to the boil, reduce the heat, cover, and cook for about 45 minutes until the barley is tender, but still with some texture, and the liquid has been absorbed. Use as required.

Porridge Measure 1 cup oats or barley flakes to 2 1/2 cups water or half milk, half water, in a non-stick saucepan. Add a little salt, if you like. Bring to the boil, reduce the heat, and simmer, stirring occasionally, for 5 minutes, or until the mixture is creamy. Alternatively, cook in a bowl in the microwave, stopping and stirring every minute.

To toast flakes or oatmeal Heat a non-stick frying pan and toss the flakes or oats over a moderate heat until golden. Do not allow to burn. Tip immediately onto a plate to cool. Store in an airtight container.

Meal suggestions (lunch only)

▸ Make a lamb or venison stew (p.51), omit the star anise and chilli and add chopped thyme and a good handful of pearl barley at the beginning.

▸ Barley cheese and vegetable soup: make a simple chunky vegetable soup with lots of root vegetables and some cabbage with a handful or pearl barley added at the beginning. When cooked, stir in some grated Cheddar or crumbled blue cheese.

▸ Cereal-coated fish or meat: mix rolled oat or barley flakes with some dried mixed herbs and a little grated onion. Season. Dip fish, pork, veal escalopes, or flattened chicken or turkey breast fillets in beaten egg, then in the cereal mixture. Fry in just a little sunflower oil for about 3 minutes on each side until golden and cooked through. Serve on wilted spinach with new potatoes and lemon wedges to squeeze over.

▸ Barley chicken salad: steam the pearl barley as before (opposite). Once cooked, fluff it up and leave to cool. Then mix with diced chicken, diced red and green peppers, drained canned sweetcorn in water, and some chopped fresh thyme. Moisten with mayonnaise flavoured with a little grated orange zest and a squeeze of the juice. Serve topped with toasted sesame seeds

▸ Make a mushroom orzotto (p.132), but substitute sliced wild or cultivated mushrooms for the winter squash and omit the cheese. Serve with a green salad.

Snack suggestions

▸ Toasted oat or barley flakes with a handful of roasted unsalted nuts and some chopped apple

▸ Toasted oatmeal stirred through natural yoghurt with some grated apple

▸ 2 oatcakes spread with houmous and topped with a slice each of cucumber and tomato

Complex carbohydrates

What to look for
• Pot barley
• Barley flakes and flour
• Oats: available rolled (porridge oats) or as coarse, medium, or fine pinhead oatmeal and bran

Ways to cook or serve
• Steam (barley)
• Loaf
• Soup
• In stews, casseroles, or hot pots
• Porridge (barley flakes and oats)
• As a coating before baking or grilling (barley flakes, oats)
• Toasted flakes or oatmeal on salads or in dips

Simple ways to flavour
• Barley goes well with root vegetables and lamb for traditional Scotch broth and in hotpots and stews.
• Toss steamed barley grains in a splash of sesame, chilli, or toasted pumpkin oil to serve as an accompaniment to meat or fish.
• Mix cooked barley with a little French dressing as a side dish with lunch.
• Mix toasted oats and barley flakes with toasted seeds and nuts and chopped fruit moistened with natural unsweetened yoghurt or milk for breakfast.

Butternut squash and blue cheese orzotto

'Orzo' means barley in Italian so this is a barley 'risotto'. Unlike risotto rice, however, this mixture remains well-textured even if you inadvertently overcook it. The result is always creamy yet nutty.

Makes 4 portions

1 small butternut squash (about 650g)
2 tbsp olive oil
1 large onion, chopped
1 garlic clove, crushed
300g pearl barley
1.2 litres strong vegetable or
    chicken stock

2 tbsp chopped fresh sage, plus a small
    handful of whole leaves
Freshly ground black pepper
6 tbsp half-fat crème fraîche
175g any blue cheese, cut into
    small pieces
A little sunflower oil

To serve: a mixed salad

1. Halve the butternut squash, scoop out the seeds, and peel. Cut the flesh into bite-sized chunks.
2. Heat the oil in a large saucepan. Add the onion and garlic and cook, stirring, for 2 minutes until softened, but not browned. Add the squash and barley and stir well. Add the stock and the chopped sage and season with black pepper. Bring to the boil, stir gently, reduce the heat, part-cover, and simmer very gently until tender with some bite and most of the liquid has been absorbed: about 40 minutes. Stir gently once or twice.
3. Gently fold in the crème fraîche and blue cheese, remove from the heat, cover, and leave to stand for 3 minutes.
4. Meanwhile make the crispy sage. Heat about 1 cm sunflower oil in a small frying pan. When really hot, but not smoking, drop in the whole sage leaves and fry for 10–15 seconds until they are bright green, start to curl and stop sizzling. Don't overcook. Remove immediately with a slotted spoon and drain on kitchen paper.
5. Spoon the orzotto onto warm plates and top with the crispy sage. Serve with a mixed salad.

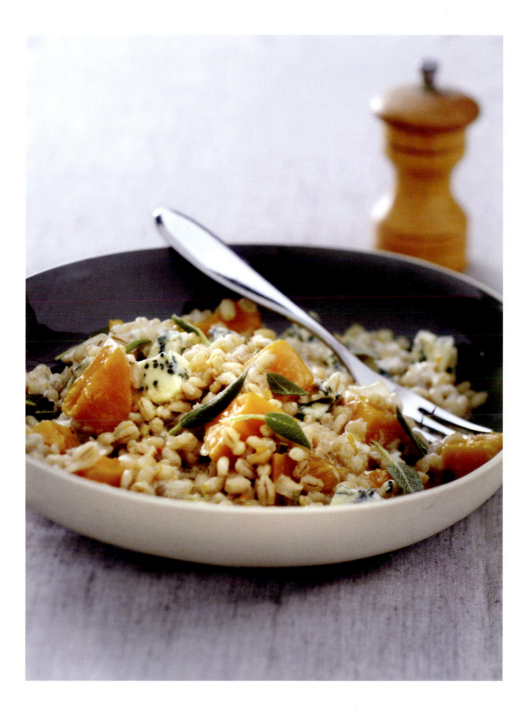

Couscous and bulgur wheat

Couscous is not a grain in itself, but is, in fact, semolina (derived from wheat) that is coated with wheat flour. Semolina does contain some protein, but is considered incomplete. It is rich in carbohydrates, and does have a high position on the glycemic index (otherwise known as high GI), therefore it could be considered to be a simple carbohydrate. However, with the addition of a protein, it makes a quick-cooking, useful contribution to your diet. Couscous is generally found pre-cooked and just requires soaking or boiling, then fluffing up with a fork.

Bulgur (bulgar/burghul) wheat is processed from a denser wheat grain and thus contains more protein and fibre, which gives it a lower score on the glycemic index (low GI). Do not confuse it with cracked wheat, which is a different product. Bulgur wheat is prepared in a similar way to couscous, but with more water and is coarser. Both keep well in an airtight container and are good store-cupboard standbys.

Three simple cooking techniques

Soak, steam, or boil Soak couscous in boiling stock or water for 5 minutes, then fluff up with a fork. It can then be steamed with other ingredients so they impart a richer flavour, if you like. Allow pretty much equal parts couscous to liquid. Bulgur wheat should be rinsed once or twice and then cooked in boiling water or stock for 15–20 minutes until the liquid is absorbed. Alternatively, soak it in the boiling liquid for 30 minutes. Then fluff up with a fork. Use 2 parts liquid to 1 part bulgur wheat.

Coating Soak as above, then flavour with herbs, spices, garlic, or grated cheese as desired and season. Dip meat, fish, chicken, halloumi cheese, firm tofu, or sliced vegetables in seasoned flour, then in beaten egg, and then in the couscous or bulgur wheat mixture. Either bake in a hot oiled roasting tin at 190°C (Gas 5), grill, or fry in just a little olive or sunflower oil, turning once until golden and cooked through.

Salad Soak as above. Add flavourings such as chopped cucumber, tomatoes, peppers, spring onions or shallots, sliced olives, nuts, seeds, diced cooked vegetables, meat, chicken, legumes, fish, cheese, herbs, spices, or garlic. Season and moisten with French dressing or olive oil and lemon juice.

Meal suggestions (lunch only)

▶ Couscous salad with halved cherry tomatoes, diced avocado, diced raw courgette, sliced red onion, chopped fresh coriander, toasted pumpkin seeds, a dash of olive and toasted pumpkin seed oils, diced halloumi cheese, black pepper, and a splash of lemon juice

▶ Couscous pilaf: add chopped cooked carrot, butternut squash, mushrooms, lamb or chicken, ground cinnamon, and black pepper to soaked couscous, heat through, and top with minted natural yoghurt

▶ Bulgur wheat salad with diced cucumber, tomato, mint, and oregano dressed with chilli oil and lemon juice, and topped with crumbled feta cheese.

▶ Tabbouleh with crushed chick-peas on lettuce: cook bulgur wheat as before (opposite) and leave to cool. Add plenty of chopped fresh mint and parsley, some finely chopped onion, and some diced cucumber and tomato and moisten with lemon juice and olive oil (this mixture also makes a good side salad). Stir in some crushed cooked chick-peas. Serve with a small dish of black olives and a separate pile of lettuce leaves: spoon some tabbouleh onto a lettuce leaf, roll up, and eat.

▶ Hot cooked bulgur wheat or couscous with chopped almonds and fresh parsley topped with a minced meat sauce (any minced meat or chicken, sautéed with a chopped onion and garlic, simmered in passata, a splash of apple juice, some chopped mushrooms, and ground cinnamon). Serve with a green salad.

Snack suggestions

▶ A spoonful of cooked couscous with a handful of chopped mixed nuts and cold cooked or raw shelled peas

▶ A spoonful of cooked couscous moistened with French dressing and spooned into a scooped-out tomato

▶ A spoonful of leftover tabbouleh with chick-peas rolled up in a lettuce leaf (above)

Complex carbohydrates

What to look for
•Couscous and bulgur wheat sold precooked. Ready-flavoured packs are also available, although avoid if they have added sugar.

Ways to cook and serve
Always cook before using
•Soak or boil
•Stir-fry
•Salad
•Side dish
•As a coating for fish or meat before sautéing or baking
•Pilaf
•Stuffing

Simple ways to flavour
•Cold with chopped fresh herbs, garlic, olive oil and lemon juice (delcious as a side salad)
•With chopped mushrooms, some chilli flakes, chopped spring onions, and oregano as a stuffing for large mushrooms, tomatoes, courgettes, peppers, or aubergines before baking
•Hot with chopped nuts or toasted seeds, olives, capers, and fresh basil as a side dish

Couscous with mint and pistachios

This is a delicious accompaniment to any spicy casserole or tagine, roast or grilled meat, or fish. Or try it topped with a couple of poached eggs and a dollop of natural unsweetened yoghurt.

Makes 4 portions

250g couscous
300ml boiling vegetable stock
55g shelled pistachios,
   roughly chopped

4 tbsp chopped fresh mint
   (or 1 tbsp dried)
Freshly ground black pepper

1. Put the couscous in a large bowl and pour over the boiling vegetable stock. Stir well, cover, and leave to stand for 5 minutes.
2. Stir in the nuts, mint, and seasoning. Put the bowl over a pan of gently simmering water, cover with a lid and steam for 10 minutes to allow the flavours to develop. Fluff up with a fork and serve hot.

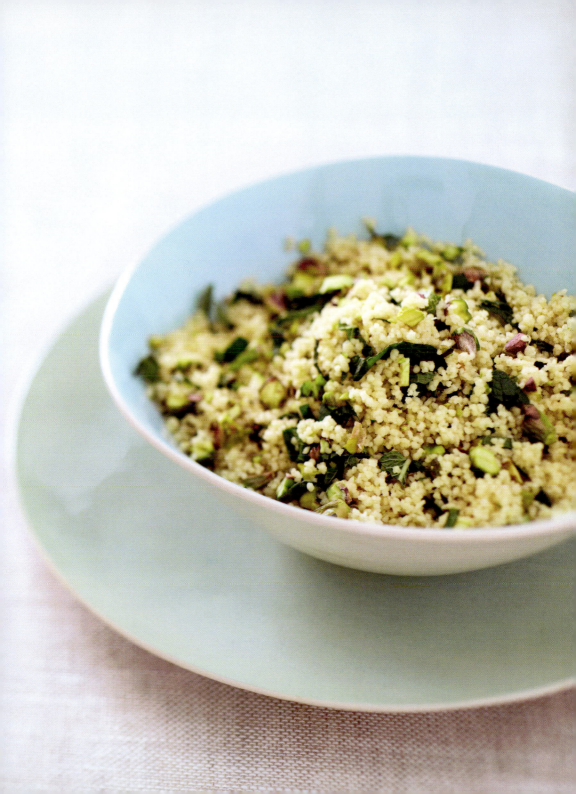

Wholewheat pasta, and buckwheat and brown rice noodles

Whole wheat is, as it sounds, made from whole grains of wheat, and as such has a high fibre content that results in a lower GI. Wheat flour is usually found in white bread and pasta and has a higher GI, as it is made from the inner part of the wheat. Wholewheat pasta has a delicious nutty flavour and texture. The pasta is usually cooked before adding to other ingredients, except when adding to soups, stews, or casseroles, which have plenty of liquid.

Despite its name, buckwheat is not a wheat, but a broadleaf plant (and not a grass, as is commonly believed). Buckwheat noodles are often sold as soba noodles. Brown rice, or udon, noodles are made from ground brown rice mixed with water. Whether dried or fresh, all pasta and noodles are an excellent way to add complex carbohydrates, texture, and interest to a meal, and they can be cooked in minutes. You can also buy wholewheat Chinese noodles in nests.

Three simple cooking techniques

Boil Add to plenty of boiling water with a pinch of salted, if you like. For spaghetti, stand the pasta in the pan and press down gently as it softens so that it bends round in the pan. Stir well, then boil for 3–4 minutes for fresh pasta, and about 10 minutes for dried, or according to the packet directions.

Stir-fry Soak or boil udon, soba, or wholewheat Chinese noodles according to the packet directions. Drain. Stir-fry meat and/or some vegetables, adding flavourings of your choice. Just before serving, add the noodles, toss, and heat through for 1 minute before serving.

Salad Cook the pasta or noodles according to the packet directions. Drain, rinse with cold water, and drain again. Tip into a salad bowl. Add chopped salad or cooked vegetables, your choice of cooked meat, poulty, fish, or cheese, and nuts or seeds, etc. Dress with mayonnaise thinned with a little olive oil and lemon juice, or French, soy sauce, or yoghurt dressing.

Meal suggestions (lunch only)

▶ Cooked udon or soba noodles tossed over a gentle heat with some crunchy peanut butter thinned with some apple juice and soy sauce, and chilli flakes, some grated lemon zest, and fresh coriander until piping hot (also good served cold)

▶ Spaghetti Bolognese: make the pasta mixture for pasta bake (p.140), spoon over cooked wholewheat spaghetti, and top with grated Parmesan or other Italian hard cheese. Serve with a green salad.

▶ Wholewheat spaghetti with broccoli and chilli, cook the pasta and add broccoli florets (or cauliflower and broccoli) for the last 5 minutes of cooking. Drain, return to the pan, add some halved cherry tomatoes, toasted sesame oil, dried chilli flakes, and toasted sesame seeds. Season and toss gently. Top with crumbled feta cheese

▶ Tuna pasta salad: cook wholewheat pasta shapes. Mix with drained, canned tuna, black olives, chopped shallot or spring onions, sun-kissed tomatoes, and diced cucumber. Dress with pesto thinned with olive oil and sharpened with lemon juice.

▶ Cook brown rice (udon) noodles in coconut milk with chopped lemon grass, some chopped red pepper, a splash of Thai fish sauce, and some Thai red curry paste. Add some chopped cooked chicken or prawns and some baby spinach leaves for the last 2–3 minutes of cooking time. Toss well.

Snack suggestions

▶ Quick chicken noodle soup: make up some chicken bouillon with good-quality concentrate or powder. Add a little chopped cooked chicken, cooked wholewheat or udon (brown rice) noodles, and cooked peas.

▶ A spoonful or two of cooked wholewheat pasta mixed with some crushed avocado, a slice or two of cooked chicken or some pine nuts, and a sprinkling of Worcestershire sauce

▶ Some cooked udon or soba noodles mixed with some coleslaw, some mixed seeds, soy beans, or fresh unsalted peanuts, and a splash of hot chilli sauce, and rolled up in a large round lettuce leaf

Complex carbohydrates

What to look for
•Wholewheat fresh and dried pasta can be found in all supermarkets as spaghetti and various pasta shapes, such as penne and rigatoni.
•Udon (brown rice), soba (buckwheat), and wholewheat Chinese noodles can be found in the speciality foods section of a supermarket.

Ways to cook or serve
•Boil
•Soup
•Stir-fry
•Side dish
•Salad
•Stew and casserole

Simple ways to flavour
•Udon, soba, and Chinese wholewheat noodles work well with sesame oil, lemon grass, chilli, and pine nuts.
•Wholewheat pasta shapes with olive oil, fresh oregano, marjoram basil or chopped rosemary, garlic and fresh Parmesan or other Italian hard cheese
•Wholewheat spaghetti with tomato-based sauces
•Toss cooked wholewheat spaghetti with tapenade, or pesto and a little olive oil, or bagna cauda (chopped, canned anchovies stirred into hot olive oil until they 'melt') with some crushed garlic and half-fat crème fraîche.

Pasta bake

This is a simple Bolognese mixture tossed with pasta, then baked in the oven with a tomato and cheese topping. Serve hot with a green salad. If you want to serve this dish in the evening, spoon the cooked meat sauce over a pile of shredded greens and sprinkle with a little grated cheese.

Makes 4 portions

2 tbsp olive oil, plus a little for greasing
1 onion, chopped
1 garlic clove, crushed
250g extra-lean minced steak
   or chicken
115g mushrooms, sliced
1 x 400g can chopped tomatoes
2 tbsp tomato purée
150ml apple juice

½ tsp dried oregano
1 tbsp soy sauce
Freshly ground black pepper
350g wholewheat penne or
   rigatoni pasta

For the topping:
2–3 largish ripe tomatoes, thinly sliced
55g Cheddar cheese, grated

To serve: a green salad

1. Heat the oil in a saucepan. Add the onion and fry, stirring, for 3 minutes until softened and lightly golden. Add the garlic and steak or chicken and fry, stirring until the meat is no longer pink and all the grains are separate.
2. Add the mushrooms, tomatoes, tomato purée, apple juice, oregano, soy sauce, and a good grinding of pepper. Bring to the boil, stirring, then reduce the heat, part-cover, and simmer gently for about 20 minutes until the sauce is rich and thick, stirring occasionally.
3. Meanwhile, cook the pasta according to the packet directions. Drain.
4. Preheat the oven to 190°C (Gas 5). Stir the cooked pasta into the sauce, then transfer the mixture to a lightly oiled 1.2-litre ovenproof dish (or 4 individual ones). Arrange the sliced tomatoes over the top and sprinkle with the Cheddar cheese. Bake in the oven for about 35 minutes until the cheese is melted, bubbling, and just turning golden. Serve hot with a green salad.

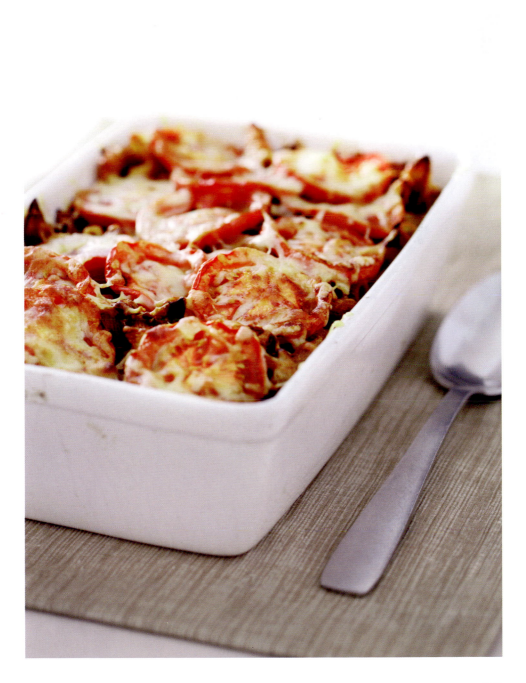

Potatoes, sweet potatoes, and yams

These tubers are related, with subtle differences. When cooked, their inherent starches turn to sugars; white potato flesh has the highest GI (glycaemic index).

There are many types of potato, from the first early, or new, potatoes with skins that rub off and small waxy potatoes to the second earlies and maincrop potatoes, which can be floury or waxy, depending on the variety. Sweet potatoes come in many sizes: smaller ones have softer skin and sweeter flesh; peel only if mashing. There are over a hundred different varieties of yam, ranging from white to orangey red inside, and they can grow enormous. The skins are rough and can be tough, so peel them unless baking them in their skins.

Potato chips and French fries are a significant source of fat and salt, but as this plan allows freedom in what you eat, fries and potato chips can be eaten as a carbohydrate very occasionally but, as always, only ever with sufficient protein.

Three simple cooking techniques

Boil Scrub or peel and cut into even-sized pieces (except for small new potatoes). Place in a pan of cold water (lightly salted, if liked). Bring to the boil, part-cover, and boil until tender (sweet potatoes cook quickest, but time will depend on sizes of chunks). Drain well.

Mash Boil as above, and drain well. Return to the pan and heat gently for a minute or two to dry out. Add a splash of milk or a spoonful of half-fat crème fraîche, if you like, and a knob of butter. Mash well with a potato masher. Alternatively, push through a potato ricer. Season with black pepper. Beat well with the masher or a wooden spoon until fluffy.

Roast Parboil (except whole new ones) in water as above, but for 2–3 minutes only. Drain. For floury peeled potatoes, cover the pan with a lid and shake vigorously to rough up the edges. Meanwhile, heat a little sunflower, nut, or olive oil in a roasting tin in the oven at 190°C (Gas 5). When hot, add the vegetables, turn over in the oil, then roast towards the top of the oven until golden and cooked through – about 45 minutes to 1 hour.

Meal suggestions (lunch only)

▸ Baked potato or sweet potato, split and topped with drained canned tuna, grated cheese, and a dollop of half-fat crème fraîche, served with a large salad

▸ Slice and layer potatoes, sweet potatoes, or yam (or a mixture) with half-fat crème fraîche, Swiss cheese, and garlic, then bake until golden. Serve on its own with salad or accompanied by roast or grilled chops, steak, chicken or fish (also good served cold, cut in wedges).

▸ Potato moussaka: layer cooked sliced potatoes with a Bolognese sauce flavoured with cinnamon. Top with thick natural unsweetened yoghurt beaten with an egg and some grated cheese. Bake at 190°C (Gas 5) until the top is set and turning lightly golden.

▸ Roast yam and sweet potato pieces with some red pepper strips, chopped rosemary, garlic, and a few dried chilli flakes, all tossed in olive oil. Top with crumbled feta cheese and serve with a green salad.

▸ Leek, yam, and lamb soup: simmer sliced leeks, diced yam, carrots, and diced lean lamb in lamb or chicken stock with some ground cumin, seasoning, and dried oregano until the lamb is tender. Add some shredded cabbage and simmer until tender.

Snack suggestions

▸ A couple of cold new potatoes with a slice of cold chicken, ham, or beef and a tomato

▸ A little cold mashed potato mixed with grated cheese and a pinch of dried mixed herbs, topped up with boiling stock and stirred for a quick soup

▸ Some diced cooked potatoes mixed with diced cucumber and a sprinkling of chopped raw peanuts moistened with mayonnaise

---

Complex carbohydrates

What to look for
•New potatoes (first earlies such as Jersey Royals) have skins that should scrape off easily with a thumb.
• Waxy salad potatoes: Charlotte and Anya (a cross between Desirée and Pink Fir Apple) are most widely available.
• Second earlies and maincrop potatoes. Maris Piper and Desirée are good all-rounders.
• Small, heavy sweet potatoes
•Firm yams without cracks

Ways to cook or serve
•Boil
•Bake
•Roast
•Sauté
•Chip
•Cooked in salad
•Mash
•Purée
•Soup
•In stews, casseroles, and curries

Simple ways to flavour
•Sauté slowly with sliced onions until caramelised (serve as a side dish or in an omelette/frittata).
•Mashed with other vegetables such as celeriac, carrots, swede, turnips, or leeks with a knob of butter or a spoonful of half-fat crème fraîche
•Cold diced pieces with mayonnaise, half-fat crème fraîche, snipped chives and some drained canned anchovies (optional) as a salad
•New boiled with a sprig of mint

Spiced wedges with garlic and herb dip

Use just one variety of tuber, if you prefer. The wedges are also great as a vegetable with grilled meat or fish served with Avocado salsa (p.183) or Sambal salad (p.189). To serve in the evening, use peeled celeriac instead, cut into thick chips.

Makes 4 portions

For the wedges:
1 small sweet potato (about 300g)
1 small yam (about 300g)
1 large potato (about 300g)
3 tbsp milk
1 tsp ground cinnamon
1 tsp ground cumin
1 tbsp sweet paprika
A few grains coarse sea salt (optional)

For the dip:
200g low-fat soft white cheese
120ml natural unsweetened yoghurt
1 garlic clove, crushed
2 tbsp chopped fresh parsley
2 tbsp chopped fresh coriander, plus
  a few torn leaves
Freshly ground black pepper

To serve:
Vegetable crudités (a selection from cherry tomatoes, radishes, sticks of carrot, cucumber, celery, sliced peppers, tiny broccoli or cauliflower florets, mangetout or sugar snap peas, baby corn cobs, raw button mushrooms, or asparagus tips)

1. Preheat the oven to 220°C (Gas 7). Scrub all three vegetables, or peel, if preferred. Cut in halves, then into thickish wedges. Toss in the milk.
2. Spread the wedges out on a large shallow non-stick baking tray (or place on baking parchment). Mix the spices together, sprinkle them all over the vegetables, and toss with your hands to coat well. Arrange the wedges on the tray so none of them overlap each other.
3. Bake in the oven for about 40 minutes, turning once until golden and crisping on the outside, and still soft in the middle. Sprinkle with just a few grains of coarse sea salt, if you like.
4. Meanwhile, make the dip. Beat all the ingredients together in a bowl, then spoon into individual pots.
5. Pile the wedges onto 4 plates, scatter with a few torn coriander leaves, and serve with the small pots of dip and plenty of crudités.

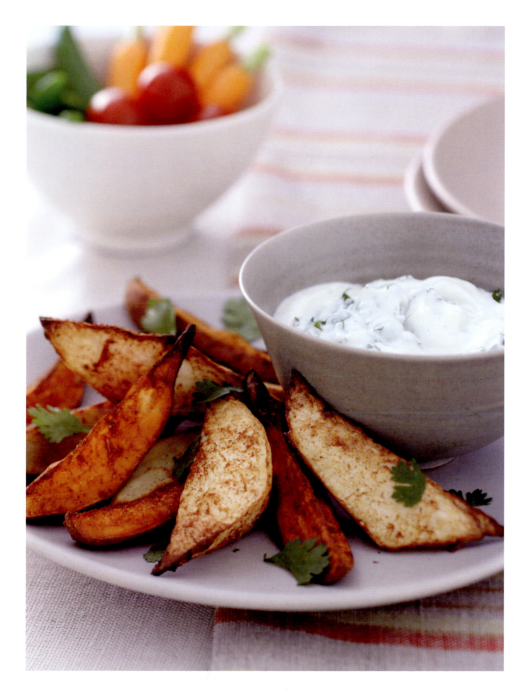

Brown rice, red rice, and wild rice
When the seeds of rice plants are hulled to remove their husks, the first layer exposed is brown – although some plants yield a red seed, or red rice. If the same seeds are milled further, the next layer, which is white, is exposed. As a result, white rice has much of its fibre and some nutrients removed, and is a refined, processed starch. This is why brown and red rice have a better fibre content than white rice.

Wild rice is a cousin of regular rice, and is classified as a grass. It has a chewy texture and takes longer to cook than brown and red rice.

Rice that is described as 'fast cook' tends to contain grains that have been milled excessively, and should be avoided as they contain little fibre.

If storing cooked rice, cool it as quickly as possible and put immediately in the fridge; if left at room temperature, it becomes a breeding ground for bacteria, which can cause food poisoning. If reheating, ensure it is piping hot before eating.

Three simple cooking techniques

Boil Bring a large pan of water to the boil. Add a pinch of salt, if you like. Add the rice, stir well, bring back to the boil, and boil for 30–50 minutes (depending on the type of rice) until just tender, but still with some 'bite' (all brown, red, and wild rices are more 'chewy' than white). This is the best way to cook wild rice.

Steam Soften a chopped onion in a little sunflower or olive oil in a pan. Add the measured amount of brown or red rice and stir until glistening. Add 21/2 times the quantity of stock or water (and any other flavouring of your choice), stir, bring back to the boil, lower the heat as much as possible, cover tightly with foil and a lid, and cook for 45 minutes. Leave undisturbed for 5 minutes, then fluff up with a fork.

Bake Prepare as for steamed rice but in a flameproof casserole. Cover and bake in a preheated oven at 190°C for 1 hour, or until tender but with some bite and the liquid has been absorbed. Fluff up with a fork.

Meal suggestions (lunch only)

- A mix of hot brown and wild rice combined with roasted vegetables as a side dish with grilled halloumi cheese, meat, or fish
- A salad of mixed Carmague red and brown rice with peppers, raw red onion, and celery moistened with a little French dressing as a side dish with grilled or roasted meat or fish
- Brown rice mixed with a chicken or tofu and vegetable stir-fry, flavoured with soy sauce and fresh ginger
- Warm salad of Camargue red rice mixed with cubes of feta cheese, cucumber, rocket, slices of spring onion, and chopped fresh herbs, and dressed with olive oil and lemon juice
- Brown rice steamed in chicken or vegetable stock with diced butternut squash. Fold baby spinach leaves through the rice when cooked so the leaves wilt, then top with a poached egg, and a dusting of grated Parmesan (or other Italian hard cheese).

Snack suggestions

- 2 heaped tablespoons of cold leftover pilaf with 2 tablespoons of drained, canned chick-peas stirred in
- 2 heaped tablespoons of cold cooked brown and wild rice with some sliced mushrooms and chopped cold chicken and spiked with lemon juice and chilli powder
- 2 bought rice cakes topped with cottage cheese and chopped chives
- 2 heaped tablespoons of cold cooked brown rice mixed with some chopped nuts, a spoonful of natural yoghurt, and some chopped fresh parsley or coriander

Complex carbohydrates

What to look for
- Choose brown basmati, long-grain, short-grain rice, and Camargue red rice.
- Wild rice is often sold mixed with brown long-grain rice, or on its own.

Ways to cook or serve
- Boil
- Steam
- Bake
- Salad

Simple ways to flavour
- Rice absorbs much of the water it is cooked in, so retains flavours well. Cooking in stock instead of water and adding a bay leaf and spices such as saffron, turmeric, cardamom pods, cinnamon, or star anise is an easy way to flavour rice to complement a main dish.
- Use tomato juice or coconut milk as an alternative to all or some of the stock or water.
- For a quick rice salad, add some chopped fresh herbs, diced cooked or raw salad vegetables, and a handful of seeds or chopped nuts, then moisten with a little French dressing.

Rice pilau with mushrooms and hazelnuts

This is a leave-to-cook dish. Use chopped or whole cashews, almonds, or raw peanuts rather than hazelnuts, if you wish. You can also serve this with a vegetable curry as well as a mixed salad.

Makes 4 portions

2 tbsp sunflower oil
1 onion, chopped
2 garlic cloves, crushed
250g chestnut mushrooms, sliced
2.5cm piece fresh root ginger, grated
300g long-grain brown rice
115g toasted hazelnuts
1 tsp garam masala

½ tsp ground coriander
750ml hot vegetable stock
1 bay leaf
Freshly ground black pepper
2 tbsp chopped fresh coriander
    or parsley
4 lemon wedges

To serve: a mixed salad

1. Heat the oil in a large saucepan. Add the onion and garlic and fry, stirring for 3 minutes until lightly golden, but not too brown.
2. Stir in the mushrooms, ginger, rice, nuts, garam masala, and ground coriander and cook, stirring, for 30 seconds.
3. Pour in the hot stock, and add the bay leaf and plenty of black pepper. Stir well and bring to the boil. Cover the pan with foil, then the lid, reduce the heat as low as possible, and cook for 45 minutes.
4. Remove from the heat and leave undisturbed for a further 5 minutes. Remove the lid, discard the bay leaf, and fluff up with a fork. Serve garnished with the chopped coriander or parsley and lemon wedges.

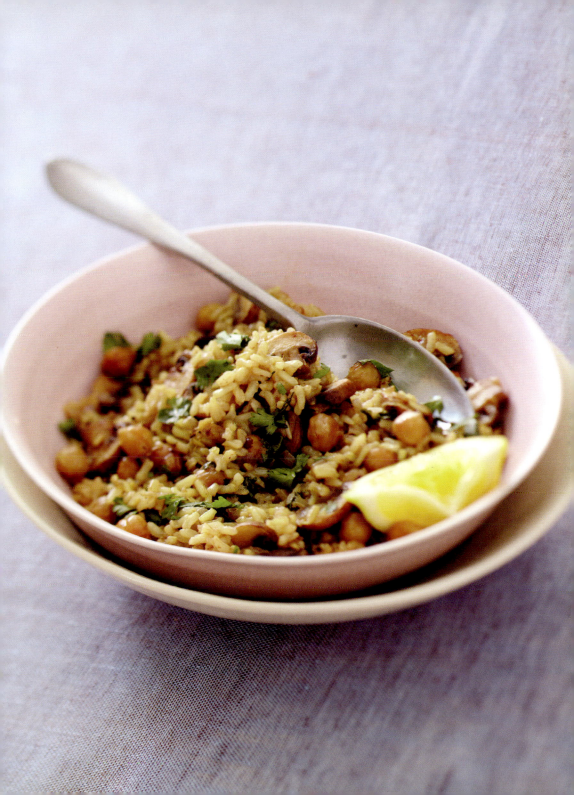

Breads

Wholegrain breads – including wholemeal bread, pumpernickel, rye bread, wholemeal pittas and chapattis, wholewheat bagels, corn and wholewheat tortillas, and Moroccan flatbreads (known as khobez) – are a staple part of the diet in most parts of the world. These wholegrain breads are a much better choice than processed white varieties.

Breads add wonderful variety to your diet, giving you the complex carbohydrates you need during the day for slow-release energy. Although you can just eat a slice of bread with your lunchtime meal, you can also do clever things with different breads, using them as receptacles for many delicious fillings or toppings.

Avoid breads that contain added sugar in the ingredients, and ensure that the amount of bread you use is matched with the right amount of protein. Thick slices of bread may look good, but it's harder to match this with an appropriate level of protein, so thin slices of bread or flatbreads are a better choice.

Three simple cooking techniques

Coating Make breadcrumbs using a blender or food processor. Leave plain or mix with flavourings such as chopped fresh herbs, spices, garlic, grated Parmesan or Cheddar cheese, or finely chopped onion. Dip raw meat, fish, chicken, halloumi cheese, tofu slices, or vegetables in seasoned flour, then beaten egg, then the breadcrumbs. Bake at 190°C (Gas 5) or sauté in a little nut or olive oil, turning once, until golden on both sides and cooked through.

Stuffing Make breadcrumbs (above). Mix with chopped herbs and/or onion, garlic, seeds, nuts, and seasoning. Mix with beaten egg to bind, then use to stuff the neck end of a chicken or other birds, escalopes of veal or pork, thin slices of beef steak, or flattened chicken breasts or turkey steaks (before rolling up), or vegetables such as peppers. Then grill, roast, or braise as required.

Bread case Cut the crusts off several large square slices of wholegrain or wholemeal bread. Dip both sides of the crusts in olive oil or a mixture of sunflower oil and melted butter. Use to line a loose-bottomed flan tin. Overlap the slices and arrange them at angles so the corners point up to give an attractive edge. Press them down well. Bake at 180°C (Gas 4) until crisp and golden brown, about 15–20 minutes. Fill as required.

Meal suggestions (for lunch only)

▶ Veal or pork escalope: coat (left) and sauté or bake (left) until golden and cooked through, turning once. Serve with lemon wedges, sautéed vine tomatoes with balsamic vinegar, green beans, and some wholewheat noodles tossed in a dash of olive oil.

▶ Ploughman's lunch: wholegrain bread with a piece of any cheese, tomatoes, cucumber, beetroot, cornichons, and pickled onions

▶ Tuna or salmon tart: make a bread case (opposite). Fill with canned tuna or salmon mixed with drained canned sweetcorn in water, and mayonnaise flavoured with tomato purée and chopped fresh herbs. Chill for 30 minutes to soften slightly before serving with a large salad.

▶ Cheese pudding: mix 2 egg yolks with 85g wholemeal breadcrumbs, 115g grated cheese, and 300ml milk. Season well and add some chopped herbs. Fold in the stiffly beaten egg whites. Tip into a greased 1.2-litre dish and bake at 200°C (Gas 6) until risen and golden. Serve with a large salad.

▶ Chicken or turkey rolls: stuff (left), simmer in chicken stock in a covered pan until tender, and serve with wilted spinach and carrots (for lunch add new potatoes).

Snack suggestions

▶ Quesadillas: put a wholemeal tortilla in a hot non-stick frying pan. Sprinkle with grated cheese (and add some grated onion or apple, if liked). Top with a second tortilla, press down, and fry until the cheese is melting and the base is crisping. Carefully tip out onto a plate, then slide it back into the pan to cook the other side, still pressing down. Cut into wedges

▶ Quick egg benedict: toast half a muffin. Top with a slice of ham, a poached egg, and then a spoonful of mayonnaise thinned with a little milk. Glaze under the grill, if you like.

▶ Vegetable rolls: put 1 or 2 cooked asparagus spears, French beans, or strips of carrot on a slice of bread (cut the crusts cut off) spread with houmous. Roll up and eat.

Complex carbohydrates

What to look for
• Wholegrain bread
• Wholemeal
• Pumpernickel
• Rye
• Wholewheat baguette
• Wholewheat English muffins
• Wholewheat pitta breads
• Wholemeal chapattis
• Wholewheat bagels
• Corn and wholewheat flour tortillas (Mexican flatbreads)
• Khobez (Moroccan flatbreads similar to tortillas, but puffy)

Ways to cook or serve
• Toast
• Bake
• Crumb coating or topping
• Baked shell (instead of pastry)
• Savoury pudding
• Stuffing

Simple ways to flavour
• Baked or toasted with olive oil or butter, garlic, and parsley for garlic bread or croutes
• Cheeses: creamy cheeses on bread topped with cress, salad leaves, or sliced beetroot; hard cheeses grated and melted on toast and topped with a sprinkling of Worcestershire sauce; white bloomed cheeses, such as goats cheese or Camembert, dipped in egg then breadcrumbs and fried in a little olive oil or brushed with oil and grilled
• Chopped fresh rosemary, black olives, walnuts or mixed seeds kneaded in wholemeal dough before shaping and baking

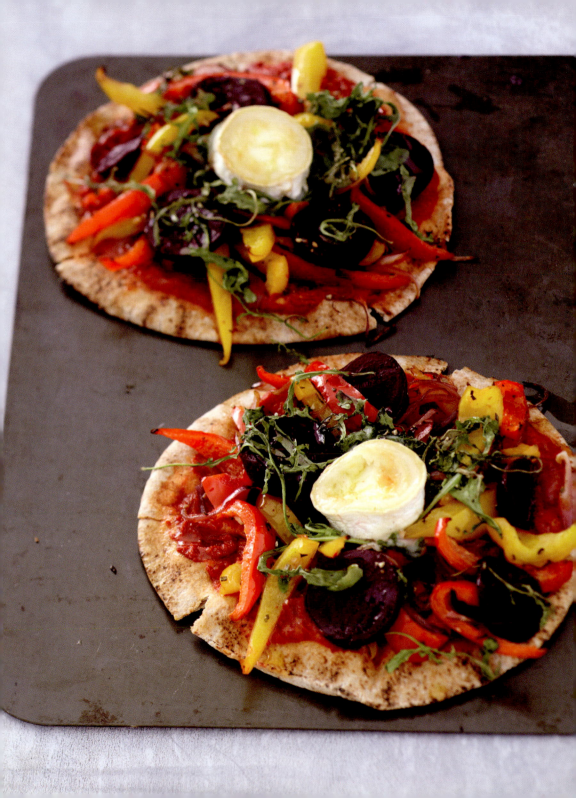

Flatbread pizza with roasted pepper, beetroot, and goats cheese

You can cheat and use a jar of pepper antipasti instead of cooking your own peppers if you prefer.

Makes 4 portions

4 tbsp olive oil
2 red and 2 yellow peppers, halved, deseeded and sliced
1 red onion, halved and thinly sliced
1 large garlic clove, finely chopped
2 tsp chopped fresh rosemary
4 wholemeal flatbreads (khobez)

4 tbsp passata (sieved tomatoes)
2 cooked baby beetroot (in natural juices), sliced
4 small handfuls wild rocket
100g disc goats cheese, sliced in 4 equal rounds
Freshly ground black pepper

1. Heat half the oil in a large saucepan or wok. Add the peppers, onion, garlic, and rosemary and cook stirring for 2–3 minutes until softening. Then cover and cook gently for 15–20 minutes until really soft, stirring occasionally.
2. Preheat the oven to 220°C. Lay the flatbreads on two baking sheets. Spread each with a tablespoon of passata, but not quite to the edges.
3. Spread the roasted peppers over the top, then scatter with the baby beetroot and rocket.
4. Put a disc of goats cheese in the centre of each flatbread. Add a good grinding of black pepper to each.
5. Bake in the oven for 5 minutes until the cheese is beginning to melt.
6. Slide onto warm plates. Drizzle each with a little of the remaining olive oil and serve straight away.

Artichokes

Part of the thistle family, artichokes are available as globe and baby artichokes. Baby artichokes are full-grown, they just come from further down the plant stalk. Once cooked, the artichoke leaves can be pulled off one by one, dipped in a sauce or dressing, and only the fleshy bases eaten (see tip, opposite). Then the little inner leaves and hairy 'choke' are cut off and the soft, succulent heart can be eaten with a knife and fork. The hearts are prepared for eating alone in this way, too, but always put them in acidulated water (vinegar or lime or lemon juice) if not cooking immediately, or they discolour. Ready-prepared artichoke hearts are also available frozen, canned, or in olive oil in jars or at the deli counter.

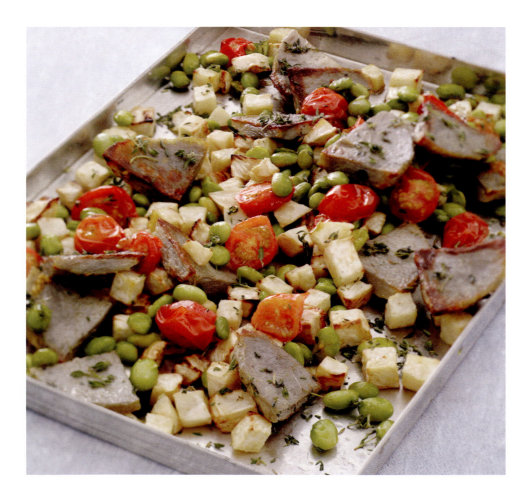

Roasted artichoke hearts with celeriac and soy beans

If you would rather not prepare fresh artichokes, use canned or frozen hearts or well-drained hearts in oil from the deli counter. Soya beans are readily available frozen, or substitute broad beans if you prefer.

Makes 4 portions

4 artichokes
1 small celeriac, peeled and cut in small chunks
4 tbsp olive oil
2 tbsp chopped fresh thyme
175g fresh or frozen soya beans
8 cherry tomatoes, halved
Freshly ground black pepper
A few coarse sea salt grains (optional)

1. Boil the artichokes in plenty of water for 20–30 minutes until a leaf pulls away easily. Drain and rinse in cold water.
2. Pull off all the leaves, cut off the stalks and hairy 'choke'. Cut each heart into quarters.
3. Preheat the oven to 200°C (Gas 6). Toss the celeriac in the oil in a roasting tray and roast in the oven for 20 minutes. Loosen with a fish slice, add the artichokes, and scatter half the thyme over. Roast for a further 20 minutes.
4. Meanwhile, boil the soya beans in a little water for 3 minutes. Drain. Add to the roasting tray with the tomatoes, drizzle with the remaining olive oil, toss gently using a fish slice, and roast for a further 10 minutes.
5. Add a good grinding of black pepper and a few grains of coarse sea salt, if you like. Scatter with the remaining thyme and serve straight away.

TIP: You could serve the leaves from fresh artichokes as a mini starter with a tiny dish of French dressing. Dip the fleshy bases into the dressing, then draw them through your teeth to eat the soft part.

Lunch only
Substitute 8 smallish new potatoes, scrubbed and quartered lengthways, for the celeriac.

Complex carbohydrates

What to look for
•The heads should be firm and tight.
•Avoid if they are open or discoloured.
•Best eaten very fresh.
•When using ready-prepared artichokes in oil, drain thoroughly before eating.

Ways to cook
•Boil (whole)
•Grill halved (baby ones or hearts)
•Roast (baby ones or hearts)
•Cooked hearts in salads
•As a pizza topping

Simple ways to flavour
•For dipping, use French dressing or melted butter, or a natural yoghurt or cheese dip.
•Grilled or roasted artichokes are good drizzled with garlic oil and grated lemon zest and juice.
•Seafood and chicken go well with the cooked hearts.

Asparagus

Although asparagus is now available in our shops all year round, local asparagus grown in season has the best flavour. Asparagus is also available frozen. Green asparagus is most common, but white asparagus is highly prized by some. It is simply regular asparagus that has been grown covered in mulch in deep trenches so is effectively grown in the dark and therefore unable to stimulate chlorophyll, the green component of vegetables.

Some people notice an unpleasant smell to their urine after eating asparagus. This is entirely normal and is simply the breakdown of sulphur-like compounds, and does not have any significance.

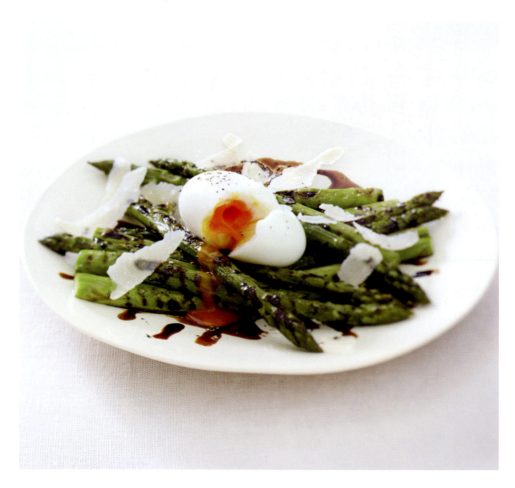

Griddled asparagus with soft-boiled eggs

This is a wonderful way to turn this most revered vegetable into a delicious light meal. Steam the spears, if you prefer, but griddling them gives them a wonderful colour and texture, and retains their full flavour. You can cheat and use bought balsamic glaze, if you prefer.

Makes 4 portions

150ml balsamic vinegar
4 or 8 eggs
675g asparagus spears
2 tbsp olive oil
30g Parmesan (or other Italian hard cheese) shavings

1. Put the vinegar in a small pan. Bring to the boil and boil rapidly until reduced by half about 1–1½ minutes. Put the base of the pan in cold water immediately to halt the cooking process, then set aside (if you reduce the vinegar too much and it gets too sticky, you can add a tiny drop more vinegar, but be careful: it will go runny again very quickly, so literally add just a drop).
2. Put the eggs in a saucepan and just cover with cold water. Bring to the boil and boil for 4 minutes. Drain and cover with cold water. When the eggs are cool enough to handle, gently tap the shells and peel them carefully.
3. Trim off about 1 cm from the base of the asparagus stalks. If they are very thick, scrape the stems with a potato peeler (but if young and fresh, this shouldn't be necessary).
4. Toss in the olive oil. Heat a griddle pan until very hot. Add the asparagus in batches and cook for 2–3 minutes, then turn over and cook for a further 2–3 minutes until just tender and striped brown. Keep warm, wrapped in foil, while you cook the remainder of the asparagus.
5. Transfer the asparagus to serving plates. Drizzle the balsamic glaze over and around the edge of the plates. Put the eggs on top of the asparagus. Scatter with a few Parmesan flakes, add a good grinding of black pepper, then gently split the eggs open so that the yolks trickle out. Serve straight away.

Lunch only
Serve with toasted wholewheat English muffins.

Complex carbohydrates

What to look for
• Choose spears with plump, firm stems that snap crisply.
• The buds at the top should be tightly closed.
• Avoid very thick stalks with woody or dirty stems.
• Best eaten very fresh, but can be stored in the chiller box in the fridge for up to 3 days
• Asparagus in oil is also found at the deli counter. Drain completely before eating.
• If you buy canned asparagus, ensure that it is in plain water without salt or sugar.

Ways to cook and serve
• Steam
• Boil
• Griddle
• Stir-fry or sauté
• Roast
• Soup
• Raw (thin tips only) or blanched in salads and as a crudités

Simple ways to flavour
• Melted butter or Hollandaise sauce with steamed or boiled spears
• Balsamic vinegar or lemon juice and olive oil for roast or griddled spears, or try chilli or lemon oil
• Eggs (soft-boiled, poached, scrambled or in a quiche, mousse, or omelette), ham (raw cured or cooked), hard or cream cheese, smoked salmon, and chicken are all favourite proteins to partner asparagus.

Aubergine

Also known as eggplant, aubergine comes in several varieties. The large, shiny, purple aubergines are the most common, although baby varieties are increasingly popular, especially in Asian cooking. Low in calories and a good 'filler' when cooked, aubergines have a creamy, soft texture and slightly sweet, almost smoky flavour. However, this vegetable does acts like a sponge, absorbing a lot of oil if you fry it, so cook in the ways suggested here to avoid adding unnecessary fat. Aubergines will keep in the fridge for several days.

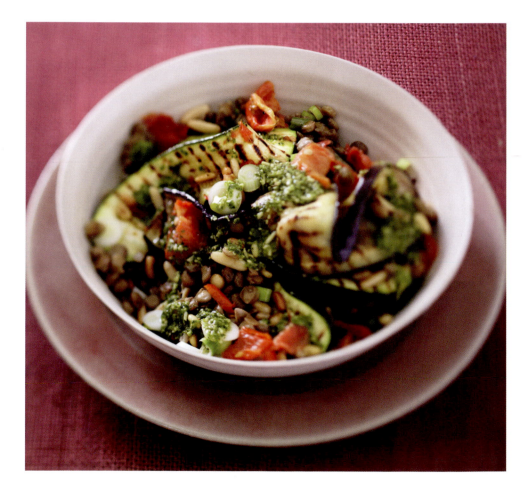

Warm aubergine, courgette, and lentil salad with pesto dressing

You can use the Rosemary and garlic pesto (p.80) for this recipe, or bought basil pesto. You can also omit the olives if you aren't keen on them. Experiment with different dried beans or chick-peas instead of lentils, too.

Makes 4 portions

1 aubergine
2 courgettes
Olive oil
55g pine nuts
2 x 410g cans of brown or green lentils, drained
   (or 450g cooked [225g raw weight] lentils)
4 spring onions, chopped
115g sun-ripened tomatoes in oil, drained, cut in bite-sized
   pieces if necessary
2 tbsp lemon juice
Freshly ground black pepper
55g black olives
3 tbsp pesto

1. Trim the aubergine and courgettes, then cut the aubergine into 8 thin slices and the courgettes into 4–6 slices lengthways. Brush all over with olive oil. Heat a griddle pan and, when hot, griddle the slices, a few at a time, for 3 minutes each side until tender and striped brown. Reheat the pan between batches.
2. Toast the pine nuts in a hot non-stick frying pan for 2 minutes or so, shaking the pan, then tip into a large bowl. Tip in the lentils and add the spring onions and the sun-ripened tomatoes. Drizzle with 2 tbsp of olive oil and the lemon juice. Add a good grinding of pepper and toss gently. Add the aubergines and courgettes and gently mix in. Carefully divide among 4 bowls, making sure each bowl gets an even amount of ingredients. Scatter the olives over.
3. Blend the pesto with a further 3 tbsp of olive oil. Spoon over the salads and serve while still warm.

Lunch only
Substitute Camargue red rice or barley for the lentils.
Bring 1.2 litres of vegetable stock to the boil in a large saucepan. Add 250g Camargue red rice (or barley), stir, bring back to the boil, reduce the heat, cover, and simmer for 30 minutes until just tender. Drain, then add the rice to the pine nuts with spring onions and tomatoes.

Complex carbohydrates

What to look for
•Aubergines should feel firm and heavy for their size.
•Press the skin, and if it leaves a dent and doesn't spring back, it's past its best.
•Avoid if the skin is wrinkly and soft, as it will taste bitter.

Healthy ways to cook
•Griddle
•Steam or boil
•Roast
•In curries, stews, and casseroles
•Purée

Simple ways to flavour
•Asian influences such as coconut milk, lemon grass, coriander, chilli, and curry pastes
•The Italian way is to griddle, cover with passata and fresh basil, top with mozzarella cheese, then grill to melt or stew with tomatoes, olives, garlic, and other Mediterranean vegetables.
•Middle Eastern spices such as cinnamon, cumin, nutmeg, and star anise, and herbs like fresh mint, parsley, and coriander with couscous or rice and/or lamb or chicken

Cabbage and leafy greens

All cabbages and leafy greens are available in one variety or another throughout the year. Baby spinach, pak choi, and red and white cabbages are good eaten raw and cooked. Swiss Chard, with white, red, yellow, or orange stems, is a two-in-one vegetable: steam the stalks and eat like asparagus, and cook the leaves as cabbage. Try Brussels sprouts shredded and stir-fried, or in soup if you don't like them boiled. Look out for lemony-flavoured sorrel and use it like spinach. Don't overcook greens and use only a little water if boiling. All are best eaten fresh, but hearty cabbages will keep much longer. Avoid storing kale for long, as it tends to become unpleasantly bitter.

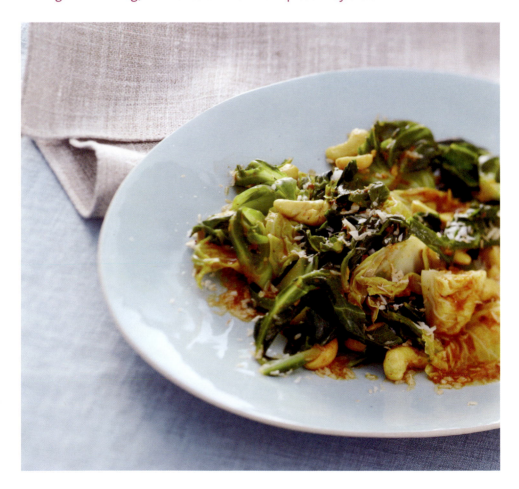

Curried spring greens
with cashew nuts

You can use any leafy greens or cabbage for this dish. It makes a meal in itself if you serve it with brown rice or chapattis for lunch, or quinoa for supper or, if you prefer, you could serve it as an accompaniment to grilled meat, chicken, or fish (in which case, omit the cashew nuts).

Makes 4 portions

450ml vegetable stock
450g spring greens, coarsely shredded, discarding thick stumps
2 tbsp mild curry paste
2 tsp lemon juice
Freshly ground black pepper
4 tbsp desiccated coconut
55g raw cashew nuts
½ tsp garam masala

1. Bring the stock to the boil in a large pan. Add the greens, stir, bring back to the boil, cover, and cook for 3 minutes until just tender. Do not overcook. Drain, reserving the stock. Put the greens to one side.
2. Pour the stock back into the pan and stir in the curry paste, lemon juice, and plenty of black pepper. Bring to the boil and boil rapidly until well reduced and slightly thickened, for about 5 minutes.
3. Meanwhile, cook the coconut in a non-stick frying pan, stirring all the time until lightly browned, for about 2 minutes. Tip it onto a plate.
4. Stir the greens, cashew nuts, and garam masala into the reduced curry sauce. Toss over a fairly high heat until piping hot. Spoon onto plates and dust with the coconut.

Complex carbohydrates

What to look for
- All varieties should be crisp and colourful; avoid if yellowing or wilting.
- For cabbages, choose firm hearty heads.

Ways to cook or serve
- Steam
- Boil
- Stir-fry or sauté
- Braise
- Stuff
- Raw in salads
- Pickle (red cabbage)
- Soup

Simple ways to flavour
- Try boiling shredded or chopped greens in a little stock instead of water, with chopped celery added.
- For stir-fried shredded greens, try ginger, garlic, lemon grass, soy sauce, chillies, and five-spice powder.
- Toasted nuts, pumpkin, coriander, cumin or sesame seeds, chestnuts, caraway, celery, and fennel seeds all add crunch and flavour.
- Shred red or white cabbage and blend with a little chopped onion, grated carrots, mayonnaise and/or thick yoghurt for fresh coleslaw.

Carrots

An inexpensive and obvious inclusion in any healthy diet, carrots also offer crunch, colour, and sweetness, and are versatile enough to be eaten cooked or raw. They are available all year, with sweet, home-grown baby and bunched carrots available from spring to autumn, and large maincrop varieties through the autumn and winter. Early spring carrots need only be scrubbed before cooking or eating raw; maincrop ones are best scraped or peeled, as the skin can be bitter. If you grow your own or buy organic carrots, shake off any excess earth, but don't wash them before storing in a cool, dark place, because they'll keep better.

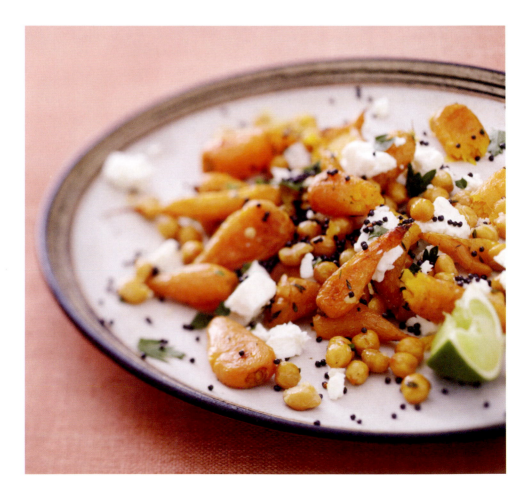

Crushed roasted carrots, chick-peas, and crumbled feta

Roasting carrots brings out their full, rich, sweet flavour. Here they're mixed with chick-peas and salty feta for extra protein, while the lovely nutty flavour of toasted black mustard seeds rounds off the dish.

Makes 4 portions

500g baby Chantenay carrots, topped and tailed
4 tbsp olive oil
1 x 410g can chick-peas in water, drained
 (or 240g cooked [115g raw weight] chick-peas)
1 tbsp chopped fresh thyme
2 tbsp black mustard seeds
115g feta cheese, crumbled
A few sprigs of flat-leaf parsley, torn
Lime wedges for garnishing

1. Preheat the oven to 190°C (Gas 5). Parboil the carrots in water for 3 minutes, then drain. Put in a roasting tin and toss in half the oil. Cover with foil and roast for 45 minutes. Add the chick-peas, sprinkle with the thyme, and roast uncovered in the oven for a further 15 minutes.
2. Roughly crush the mixture with the back of a wooden spoon (but not too much). Transfer to a warm shallow serving dish.
3. Heat the remaining olive oil in a small frying pan. Add the mustard seeds and heat until they begin to 'pop'. Pour the oil and seeds over the carrots and chick-peas.
4. Scatter the feta and a few torn flat parsley leaves over the top and serve warm with lime wedges.

Lunch only
Add warm wholemeal pitta bread.

Complex carbohydrates

What to look for
• Darker-coloured carrots (which have higher levels of nutrients and flavour)
• Bunched carrots (twist off the stalks before storing, or they'll quickly go limp)
• Avoid wet carrots. If you have to buy washed ones, store them in the fridge.

Ways to cook or serve
• Steam
• Boil
• Stir-fry
• Soups
• Stews and casseroles
• Roast
• Juice
• Raw (grated for salads and snacks or in sticks for crudités)

Simple ways to flavour
• Grated orange zest and juice: add to carrot soup or when stir-frying carrots for added zing.
• Seeds (for delicious nuttiness): roasted sesame, mustard, celery, fennel, or sunflower seeds
• Sweet spices: add smoked paprika, cumin, coriander, ginger, or cinnamon to soups, stews, casseroles, and stir-fries containing carrots.
• Roasted with other roots such as beetroot, celeriac, and parsnip
• Mashed with potatoes, celeriac, butternut squash, pumpkin, or swede

Flowering greens

This group includes varieties of broccoli and cauliflower, and romanesco, which is similar but with a really pretty, spiked lime-green head. Cauliflowers aren't just available with creamy white florets, orange and purple varieties are now grown, too. Calabrese is the Italian name for broccoli and it has a tight cluster of small green heads. Purple, and white, sprouting broccoli, on the other hand, sprout many heads from one long stalk, which are cut separately. Cook all of these varieties as lightly as possible to avoid that unpleasant sulphurous smell that can permeate everywhere and to retain maximum nutrients.

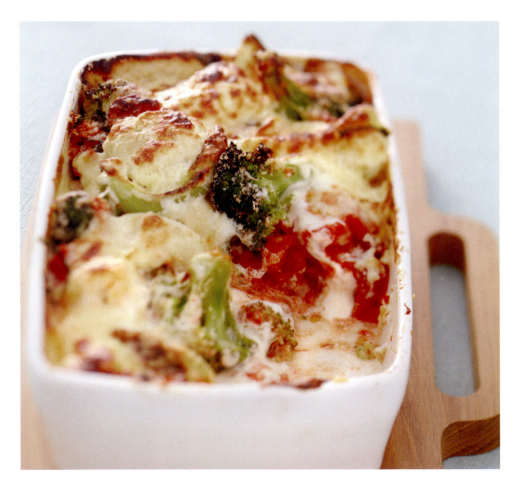

Broccoli, cauliflower, and tomato cheese bake

This is a very simple version of a traditional cauliflower cheese, but with no complicated sauce to make. It makes a complete meal with the addition of some warm wholegrain bread, or use in half-sized portions as a side dish for grilled fish or chicken.

Make 4 portions

1 small cauliflower
1 broccoli head, about 350g
2 ripe beefsteak tomatoes
2 tbsp tomato purée
Freshly ground black pepper
2 tbsp chopped fresh basil
400ml half-fat crème fraîche
115g strong Cheddar cheese, grated
55g Parmesan or other Italian hard cheese, grated

1. Preheat the oven to 190°C (Gas 5). Cut the cauliflower and broccoli into even-sized florets, discarding the thick stump. You can tear off any green leaves from the cauliflower stalks to cook with the florets, if you like.
2. Cook the vegetables in boiling water for 3–4 minutes until just tender but still with some 'bite'. Drop the tomatoes in for the last minute, then quickly remove with a slotted spoon and put in a bowl of cold water. Drain the cauliflower and broccoli thoroughly and tip into a 1.5-litre ovenproof serving dish.
3. Peel the skin off the tomatoes and chop the flesh. Mix with the tomato purée, then spoon over the cooked vegetables. Season with black pepper and scatter over the chopped basil.
4. Mix the crème fraîche with the Cheddar cheese and spoon over. Sprinkle the top with the grated Parmesan cheese. Bake in the oven for 40–45 minutes until golden. Serve hot.

Lunch only
Mix 55g wholemeal breadcrumbs with 1 tbsp olive oil and the Parmesan and scatter over the top of the dish before baking.

Complex carbohydrates

What to look for
•Cauliflowers and romanesco should all have tight, firm heads. Avoid if discoloured, they smell strong, are beginning to bolt, or if florets have obviously been trimmed to cut off blemishes.
•Calabrese should be firm, not floppy, and uniformly green. Avoid heads with long stalks.
•Choose sprouting broccoli with thin stems that snap crisply. Avoid purple-sprouting with flecks of yellow – it's past its best (don't confuse white-sprouting with yellowing purple-sprouting broccoli).

Ways to cook or serve
•Steam
•Boil (lightly)
•Stir-fry or sauté
•Soup
•Tiny florets raw as crudités
•Pickle (cauliflower)

Simple ways to flavour
•Cheese tossed with the cooked vegetables or as a coating sauce
•Lightly cooked florets with flaked almonds, lemon juice, chilli, garlic, and olive oil on their own, or tossed with wholewheat spaghetti or udon noodles
•Mix with curry pastes or dress with chopped tomatoes, hard-boiled egg, toasted oatmeal, and plenty of parsley or coriander.

Pods and beans

This group incorporates all the podded vegetables we eat, including the pods. It includes small French (green) beans, the longer, flat Helda and runner beans, mangetout, and sugar snap peas.

The best-flavoured runner beans are home-grown, but the majority are imported and are available pretty much all year. They require varying degrees of preparation. French beans, mangetout, and sugar snap peas just need topping and tailing. French beans can then be cut into chunks, if liked. Helda beans should be topped and tailed and cut into chunks or diagonal slices; runner beans need the strings to be cut off all round and then cut in diagonal slices or diamonds.

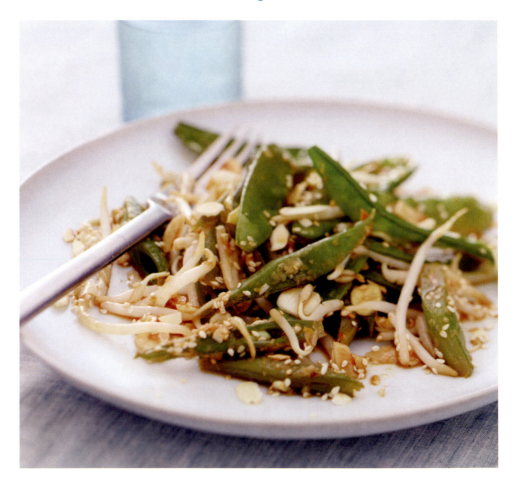

Stir-fried green beans and mangetout

Use French beans, cut in short lengths, instead of runner or Helda beans, if you prefer, and try using sugar snap peas instead of mangetout. This recipe makes a light lunch rolled up in wholewheat bread wraps, but is also really good served with grilled or stir-fried fish, chicken, beef, or pork (with some wholewheat Chinese noodles, if serving at lunchtime).

Makes 4 portions

4 tbsp sesame seeds
4 tbsp flaked almonds
350g runner or Helda beans
2 tbsp sunflower oil
4 spring onions, cut in short lengths
115g mangetout
115g pea or bean sprouts
1 large garlic clove, crushed
2.5cm piece fresh root ginger, grated
2 tbsp rice-wine vinegar
3 tbsp soy sauce
1 tbsp sesame oil

1. Heat a small frying pan and quickly toast the sesame seeds and almonds, stirring for about 2 minutes until turning golden. Tip out onto a plate and reserve.
2. If using runner beans, trim them all the way round to cut off the stringy edge. If using Helda beans, just top and tail them. Cut the beans in diagonal slices.
3. Heat the sunflower oil in a wok or large frying pan. Add the beans, spring onions, and mangetout and stir-fry for 4 minutes until softening.
4. Add the remaining ingredients, including half the sesame seeds and almonds, and toss for a further 2 minutes. Serve straight away, sprinkled with the remaining sesame seeds and almonds.

Complex carbohydrates

What to look for
• The pods should be firm and snap easily when bent.
• They should be bright green; avoid if they look grey or shrivelled.
• Avoid thick large beans, as they will be tough.
• When trimming runner beans, discard any you can't cut easily, as they will be stringy when cooked.
• Frozen beans are equally as nutritious as fresh.
• If buying canned beans, choose varieties in water with no added sugar or salt.

Ways to cook or serve
• Steam
• Boil
• Stir fry
• Blanched in a salad (French beans only)

Simple ways to flavour
• Dress with olive oil and black pepper and sprinkle with toasted almonds or pine nuts.
• For hot or cold French beans, add walnut oil or toasted sesame oil, finely chopped onion or shallot, and lemon juice.
• Stir soft white cheese thinned with milk and flavoured with plenty of chopped fresh herbs through beans before serving.
• Ginger, chilli, soy sauce, and a splash of apple juice

Sweetcorn, shelled peas, and broad beans

These starchy little vegetables are interchangeable in many dishes. They all have distinctive flavours, but also add colour and texture. Fresh peas and cut corn kernels can be eaten raw, but broad beans should always be cooked. Unless very young, the skins of broad beans can be tough, so it's best to pop them off after cooking and before serving. Sweetcorn can be eaten whole on the cob or as the kernels cut off. To do this, simply hold the cob upright on a board and slice downwards with a sharp knife all round the cob. Corn on the cob must be eaten very fresh. Baby corn is just immature ears harvested as soon as the silks appear.

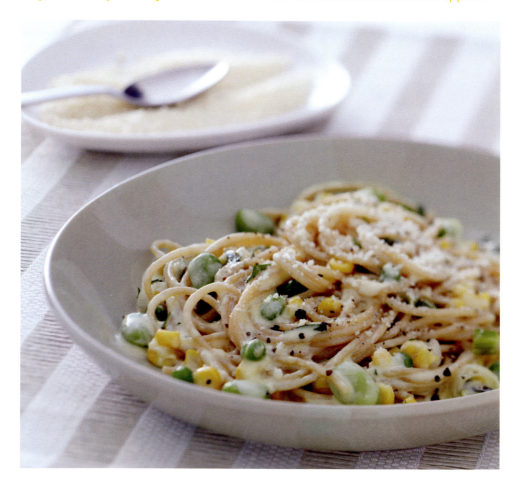

LUNCH ONLY   # Vegetable carbonara

This recipe is a delicious lunch dish when you have the time to cook and enjoy it. You could try tossing it through lightly steamed vegetable ribbons or shredded leeks to serve it in the evening.

Makes 4 portions

2 fresh ears of corn or 115g frozen corn kernels
175g shelled fresh or frozen baby broad beans
175g fresh or frozen soya beans
2 tbsp sunflower oil
1 bunch of spring onions, chopped
2 garlic cloves, crushed
115g shelled fresh or frozen peas
350g wholewheat spaghetti
2 tbsp chopped fresh parsley
1 tbsp chopped fresh mint
2 eggs
200ml half-fat crème fraîche
55g Parmesan or other Italian hard cheese, grated
Freshly ground black pepper

1. If using fresh corn, cut the kernels off the cobs (opposite).
2. Cook the broad beans and soya beans in a little boiling water for 5 minutes and set aside.
3. Heat the oil in a small pan, add the spring onions and garlic, stir, cover, reduce the heat, and cook very gently for 5 minutes. Add the corn and peas, stir, cover, and cook very gently for a further 3 minutes.
4. Meanwhile, cook the spaghetti according to the packet directions. Drain and return to the pan.
5. Add the pea and corn mixture, the cooked beans, the parsley, and mint. Whisk the eggs with the crème fraîche and half the Parmesan. Pour into the pan. Add a good grinding of pepper.
6. Toss over a very gentle heat until hot through and creamy. Do not allow the eggs to scramble. Taste and re-season, if necessary. Pile onto warm plates and sprinkle with the remaining cheese.

Complex carbohydrates

What to look for
• Corn on the cob: choose plump cobs with creamy pale yellow kernels. The darker the colour, the more the sugar will have turned to starch, so the corn won't be so sweet.
• Broad beans: choose soft pods with beans no bigger than a thumbnail for best eating (older beans have a very floury texture and tough skins.
• Peas: pick bright-green full pods, but with a tiny space still between the peas. If the pods look dry, discoloured, and fit to burst, the peas are over-mature, hard, and floury, and not sweet.

Ways to cook or serve
• Boil
• Steam
• Grill (for corn on the cob)
• Stir-fry
• Salad (and baby ears as crudités)
• In pasta and rice dishes
• Side dish
• Soup
• Stews, curries, and casseroles

Simple ways to flavour
• Peas with mint are a classic combination.
• Lean raw cured or cooked ham added to any beans with some sautéed chopped onion, garlic, and crème fraîche (on their own or stirred through spaghetti)
• Cheddar and other hard cheese with sweetcorn in chowder, sauce, or melted over cobs

Onions and leeks

The tasty, distinctive flavour of onions and leeks means they can be eaten on their own or used to add depth to just about any savoury dish. Onions come in many varieties – red, white, brown, baby, large, sweet, shallots, spring, and salad – and all are good choices. Freezing an onion for 30 minutes or so before chopping it can reduce the effects of the sulphur-like compound that affects the eyes and induces tears. Onions are available all year round, fresh or from store, and frozen chopped onion is a great convenience food to have. Leeks are a milder alternative to onions, both raw in salads and cooked. Look out for baby leeks, too, which are delicious cooked whole and served hot or cold.

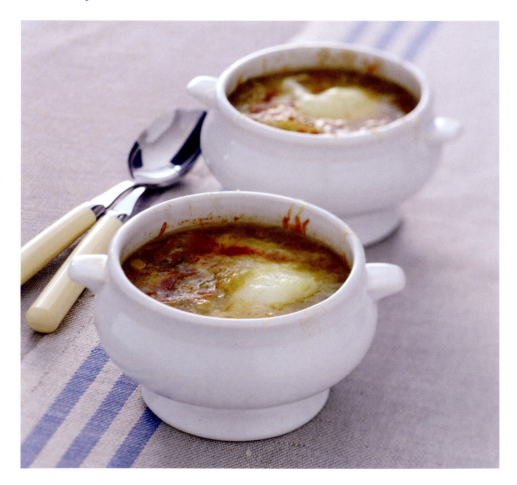

French leek and onion soup with poached eggs

You can use all leeks or all onions for this, if you prefer, but you get a lovely depth of flavour using a combination of both. It's worth making double the quantity of the soup base and either keeping it in the fridge for a few days or freezing it for a future occasion.

Makes 4 portions

3 tbsp sunflower oil
2 fairly large onions (about 350g total weight), halved and sliced
2 large leeks, well-washed and sliced
4 tbsp quinoa
1 litre strong beef or vegetable stock
1 bay leaf
Freshly ground black pepper
4 eggs
85g Gruyère or Cheddar cheese, grated

1. Heat the oil in a large saucepan. Add the onions and leeks and fry, stirring until they begin to soften and colour, for about 4 minutes. Then reduce the heat as low as possible, cover, and cook very gently for 10 minutes. Remove the lid, turn up the heat, and fry, stirring for 3–4 minutes until golden. Stir in the quinoa.
2. Add the stock, the bay leaf, and some seasoning. Bring to the boil, reduce the heat, cover, and simmer gently for 20 minutes.
3. Preheat the grill. Break the eggs, one at a time, into a cup and slide each into the simmering soup. Cover and simmer for 2–5 minutes, depending on how well-cooked you like your eggs. Carefully lift out the eggs with a slotted spoon and place in 4 flameproof deep soup bowls (don't worry if there are odd bits of egg white left behind). Ladle the soup over.
4. Cover the top of each bowl with the grated cheese and place under the grill until melted and bubbling, about 3 minutes.

Lunch only
Serve with wholemeal baguette.

Complex carbohydrates

What to look for
• Chose firm, round onions with dry, papery outer skins. Avoid any with a strong smell or if wet.
• Spring and salad onions should have bright-green tips and look crisp and juicy.
• Avoid very dirty leeks. Always trim them first and then wash thoroughly, as they may be full of dirt and grit.
• Pickled onions are acceptable, but bear in mind that they can be a significant source of salt, and possibly sugar as well.
• Store salad onions and leeks in the fridge wrapped in a plastic bag to prevent the smell permeating other foods. Store onions in a cool, dark place.

Ways to cook
• Stir-fry or sauté
• Sauce
• Raw (or steamed whole baby leeks) in salads and sandwiches
• Soups
• Stews, curries, and casseroles
• Roast
• Stuffed (large ones)

Simple ways to flavour
• With tomatoes: either raw in salads or sandwiches, or cooked for sauces or soups, or finely chopped as a salsa with chopped coriander moistened with lime juice and olive oil
• With cheeses of all sorts
• As a marinade with either sage rosemary, thyme, oregano, or basil and oil and lemon juice

Squashes

With their wonderful bright colours and tasty, slightly nutty flavoured flesh, squashes are good on their own as an accompaniment to a main dish or as an ingredient to enrich many dishes. Tender, creamy-fleshed, immature summer squashes include long green, yellow, and crook-neck courgettes, the round 'ball' courgettes, and patty-pan squashes. Baby varieties to cook whole are also available. There are also hard-skinned winter varieties with more fibrous flesh and a sweet flavour, such as pumpkin, marrow, and spaghetti, butternut, acorn, harlequin, gem, and onion squashes.

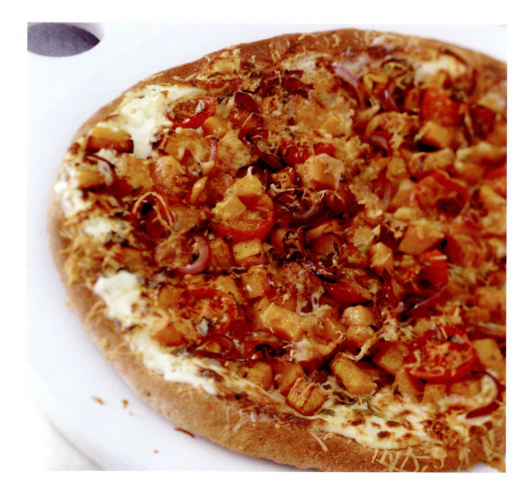

LUNCH ONLY

Roasted pumpkin and red onion pizza

This is a lunchtime treat, although the topping can be used as a stuffing for peppers for an evening meal.

Makes 2–4 portions

For the pizza dough:
225g strong wholemeal bread flour
15g Parmesan (or other Italian hard cheese), grated
2 tsp easy-blend dried yeast
1 tbsp olive oil
2 tbsp milk
For the topping:
4 tbsp olive oil
1 large red onion, halved and sliced
2 garlic cloves, chopped
½ small pumpkin or butternut squash (about 350g), peeled, deseeded, and cut into smallish chunks
4 tbsp low-fat white soft cheese
6 baby plum or cherry tomatoes, halved
2 tbsp chopped fresh sage
55g Edam cheese, grated
75g buffalo mozzarella, thinly sliced
Freshly ground black pepper
A few grains coarse sea salt (optional)

1. Mix the flour, cheese, and yeast in a bowl. Add the oil, milk, and 150ml warm water. Mix to form a soft but not sticky dough. Knead gently on a lightly floured surface for 5 minutes until smooth and elastic. Place back in the bowl, cover with oiled cling film, and leave in a warm place for 1 hour, or until doubled in bulk.
2. Meanwhile, heat half the oil in a large saucepan. Add the onion and cook, stirring, for 2 minutes until softened but not browned. Add the garlic and pumpkin. Stir well, cover, and cook gently for 10 minutes until just tender, stirring once. Set aside.
3. Preheat the oven to 220°C (Gas 7). Place a large baking sheet or pizza pan in the oven to heat. When the dough has risen, knock back, re-knead, and roll out to a 30cm round. Oil the hot baking sheet or pan and put the dough on it.
4. Quickly spread the white soft cheese over the dough. Spread the onion and squash mixture over and scatter over the tomatoes, sage, and cheeses. Season and drizzle with the remaining oil.
5. Bake in the oven for 20 minutes or until the bread is crisp and brown round the edges and the cheese is melted and bubbling. Sprinkle with a few grains of sea salt, if you like, and serve hot.

Complex carbohydrates

What to look for
• Summer squashes should have shiny skin, be fairly small and firm, and the skin should pierce easily with your fingernail.
• All squashes should feel heavy for their size.
• Winter squashes should have hard skin.

Ways to cook
Summer squash:
• Steam
• Stir-fry or sauté
• Griddle
• Stuff
• Soup
• Raw, grated in salads, sticks for crudités
Winter squash:
• Soup
• Roast
• Purée
• Stuffed

Simple ways to flavour
• Nutmeg, cinnamon, and ginger go well with pumpkin and other really sweet winter squashes for purees and roasted pieces.
• Sautéed sliced courgettes are good with olive oil, garlic, lemon juice, dill, and fennel seeds.
• Tomatoes, onions, cheese, or a Bolognese mixture make a good stuffing for marrow rings or halved larger courgettes, or try them coated in cheese sauce.
• Try a savoury custard flavoured with herbs baked in the cavities of butternut or acorn squashes.

Other root vegetables

Root vegetables such as turnips, swede, parsnips, and beetroot are all hardy, nutritious, and easy to use in a variety of ways. This group also includes kohlrabi, which is technically part of the cabbage family and is a swollen stem, but is prepared and eaten like turnip. These vegetables all have varying depths of sweet, earthy flavour and can enhance all sorts of savoury dishes, as well as being delicious cooked and eaten on their own as a side dish or even thinly sliced or grated and served raw when very fresh. Remember, if cooking beetroot, not to cut into the flesh before boiling it or the colour will 'bleed'. It's best to wear rubber gloves when peeling beetroot to protect your fingers from staining.

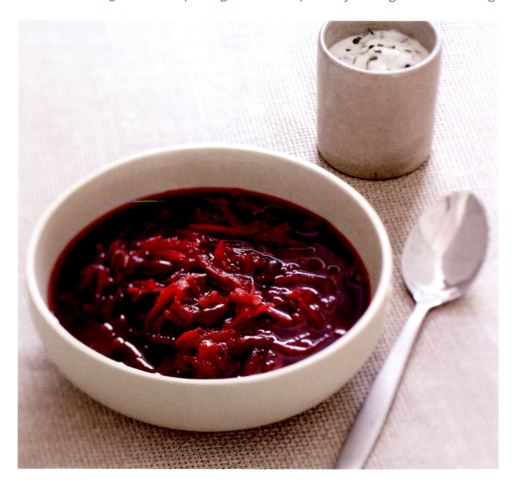

Mixed root and red bean borscht with chive yoghurt

This hearty soup makes a delicious lunch or supper dish – with big portions. You can use other beans, if you prefer, or try it with chick-peas, too.

Makes 4–6 portions

1 turnip or small kohlrabi
¼ swede
1 small parsnip
2 large beetroot
1 red onion
1 celery stick
1 x 410g can red kidney beans in water, rinsed and drained
    (or 240g cooked [115g raw weight] beans)
1.2 litres strong vegetable stock
3 tbsp red-wine vinegar
1 bay leaf
A good pinch of ground cloves
Freshly ground black pepper
4–6 tbsp thick natural yoghurt
2–3 tbsp snipped chives

1. Coarsely grate all the vegetables. Place in a large saucepan and add the beans.
2. Stir in the stock, vinegar, bay leaf, cloves, and a good grinding of black pepper. Bring to the boil, part cover, reduce the heat, and simmer gently for 30 minutes or until the vegetables are really tender. Discard the bay leaf.
3. Meanwhile, mix the yoghurt with the chives and set aside.
4. When the soup is cooked, taste and re-season, if necessary. Ladle into warm bowls and serve topped with the chive yoghurt.

Lunch only
Serve with pumpernickel bread.

Complex carbohydrates

What to look for
•Root vegetables should feel heavy for their size.
•Avoid the largest specimens, as they will be fibrous, not so sweet, and hard to cut up.
•Remove beetroot leaves immediately (and cook them like spinach), as the roots will stay fresh longer.
•Store in a cool, dark place

Ways to cook or serve
•Steam
•Boil
•Roast
•Mash
•Purée
•Raw in salads
•Soups, stews, and casseroles
•As a topping instead of – or mixed with – potato

Simple ways to flavour
•Cumin, coriander, dill, caraway, and mustard seeds, or chopped walnuts are good sprinkled over roots once steamed, or before roasting in a little olive oil.
•Beat crème fraîche and some chopped fresh parsley into a root purée or mash for a deliciously moist side dish with grilled meat or fish.
•Grate and mix with a little olive oil, white balsamic, black pepper, and snipped chives for a simple salad.
•Top boiled or steamed small cubes with a dollop of natural yoghurt, crumbled feta cheese, and finely chopped spring onions

Peppers

Nutritious and versatile, peppers add colour, flavour, and texture to salads, main meals, and side dishes. The most familiar varieties are large bell-shaped capsicums that are usually green, yellow, orange, or red (and sometimes purple or white) and have a distinctive sharp flavour and varying degrees of sweetness. Look out, too, for ramiro or romano peppers, which are long, flat, and much sweeter. Hotter chilli peppers are smaller in size, ranging from fat jalapeños and round Scotch bonnets to tiny, thin birds-eye chillies, and their heat ranges from mild to mouth-numbing. After deseeding and slicing chillies, wash your hands carefully, as chilli juice is potentially very irritating to the skin.

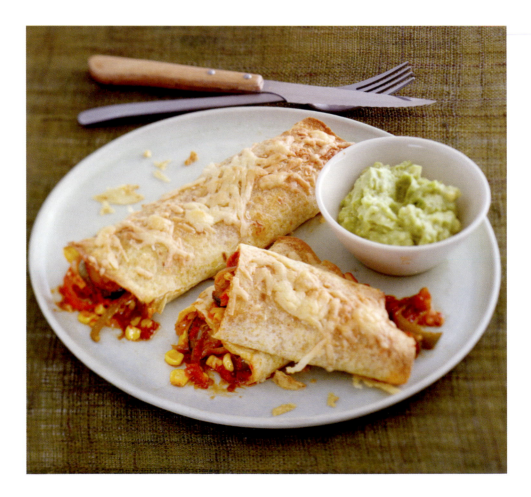

LUNCH ONLY

Mixed pepper enchiladas with guacamole

For a quicker dish, simply warm the tortillas, fill with the pepper mixture, add grated cheese, a little guacamole, and a spoonful of half-fat crème fraîche, roll up, and eat.

Makes 4 portions

1 fresh ear of corn or 55g frozen sweetcorn
2 tbsp olive oil
1 large onion, halved and sliced
2 red and 2 green peppers, halved, deseeded, and sliced
1 courgette, sliced
2 tsp ground cumin
¼ tsp dried chilli flakes
1 tsp dried oregano
4 tomatoes, chopped
2 tbsp tomato purée
Freshly ground black pepper
8 corn tortillas
410g can red kidney beans, rinsed and drained
  (or 240g cooked [115g raw weight] beans), mashed
115g Cheddar cheese, grated
For the guacamole:
2 ripe avocados
Juice of 1 lime

To serve: a crisp salad

1. Preheat the oven to 190°C (Gas 5). Cut the corn off the cob if using fresh corn (p.168). Heat the oil in a large frying pan or wok. Add the onion and fry for 2 minutes, stirring until softened but not browned. Add the peppers and courgettes and fry, stirring, for 5 minutes until fairly soft.
2. Add the spices and fry for 30 seconds. Stir in the sweetcorn, oregano, tomatoes, and tomato purée, cover, and cook, stirring occasionally, for a further 5 minutes, or until tender. Season with freshly ground black pepper.
3. Divide the mixture among the tortillas, top each with a spoonful of mashed beans, roll up, and pack into a shallow ovenproof dish. Sprinkle liberally with the grated cheese. Bake in the oven for about 35 minutes until the top is bubbling and lightly golden and the tortillas are crisp at the edges.
4. Meanwhile, make the guacamole. Halve the avocados and scoop out the flesh into a bowl. Mash well with a fork, then beat in the lime juice. Serve the enchiladas hot with the guacamole.

Complex carbohydrates

What to look for
•Choose firm, shiny specimens.
•Green peppers have the sharpest flavour, and go through varying degrees of ripeness to red (the sweetest).
•Avoid any that have soft spots or appear shrivelled.
•Choose chillies carefully. As a general rule, large, fatter ones are milder than tiny thin ones but it isn't always the case. Scotch bonnet, or habanero, chillies are seriously hot!

Ways to cook or serve
•Stuff
•Roast
•Salad
•Stir-fry or sauté
•Stew and casserole
•Soup
•Sauce

Simple ways to flavour
•Olive oil, garlic, red onions, and chopped fresh rosemary for roast or sautéed peppers
•Romano or ramiro or large flat chillies stuffed with soft white cheese, or goats cheese, and grilled
•Tomatoes, onions, garlic, and olives with fresh oregano, basil, or thyme
•Peppers also complement eggs, chicken, beef, veal, and fish.

Mushrooms

There are a wide variety of cultivated and wild mushrooms to enjoy. If you are going to forage for wild mushrooms, and you are not sure about different varieties, go with a guide. If in doubt, don't pick them. Mushrooms have varying degrees of flavour, ranging from the more familiar delicate earthiness of button mushrooms to the nutty richness of shiitake mushrooms. Combining mushroom varieties is a good way to enjoy their different flavours and textures. Most just need wiping before use; only peel large, flat field mushrooms, which may have tough skins.

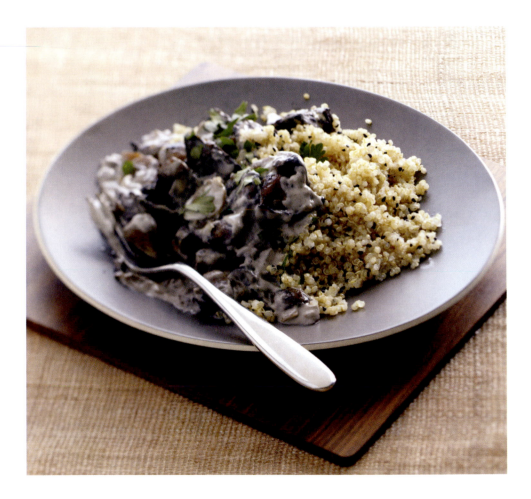

Mushroom and chestnut stroganoff

You can use fresh chestnuts if you have time to prepare them. Nick the skins, put them in a bowl, and cover with boiling water. Leave for 5 minutes. Lift them out one at a time and, with rubber-gloved hands, remove the shell and inner skin. Then boil until just tender.

Makes 4 portions

4 tbsp sunflower oil
1 onion, chopped
2 garlic cloves, crushed
675g mushrooms, quartered
1 x 200–240g can or vacuum pack of chestnuts, halved
150ml vegetable stock
2 tbsp white balsamic
400ml half-fat crème fraîche
Freshly ground black pepper
250g quinoa
2 tbsp black onion seeds
A little chopped fresh parsley

To serve: a mixed salad

1. Heat 2 tbsp of the oil in a large pan and fry the onion fairly gently for about 5 minutes, stirring until golden.
2. Add the garlic and mushrooms. Cover and cook gently for 10 minutes. Remove the lid and continue cooking for a minute or 2 until all the liquid has evaporated, stirring occasionally.
3. Add the chestnuts, stock, and balsamic condiment and simmer gently, uncovered, for about 5 minutes until nearly all the liquid has evaporated.
4. Stir in the crème fraîche and season with black pepper.
5. Meanwhile, cook the quinoa according to the packet directions. Drain. Heat the remaining 2 tbsp oil in the quinoa pan. When the oil is hot, add the onion seeds and cook, stirring, until they start to 'pop'. Return the quinoa to the pan and toss until every grain is coated in the oil.
6. Spoon the quinoa onto warm plates and top with the stroganoff. Sprinkle with a little chopped parsley and serve.

Lunch only
Substitute 250g wholewheat tagliatelle for the quinoa.

Complex carbohydrates

What to look for
Some common varieties:
• Cup (closed and open), white or chestnut: everyday mushrooms to cook whole or sliced
• Large flat (white, portabello): stronger flavour
• Oyster (various colours): mild flavour, fan-shaped
• Shiitake: meaty-textured and good flavour
• Chanterelle: yellow or orange trumpet shape; also sold dried
• Morel: one of the most sought after, with a dark, honeycomb, hooded top, and delicious flavour, often sold dried
• Cep or porcini: meaty and well-flavoured. Often sold dried
• Field: common wild mushroom. The bigger the better for taste

Ways to cook or serve
• Sauté
• Bake
• Stir-fry
• Salad
• Soup
• Stuff
• Pâté
• Risotto

Simple ways to flavour
• Sautéed in garlic and butter and olive oil with fresh parsley
• Baked in garlic and cream with a splash of apple juice
• With raw cured or cooked ham eggs, and/or tomatoes
• Cumin, coriander seeds, chilli, oregano, thyme, and bay leaves all add great flavour.

Jerusalem artichokes and celeriac These may
seem odd bedfellows, but they are both unusual vegetables that can be cooked in many of the same ways. Jerusalem artichokes are members of the sunflower family. They are knobbly tubers with a distinctive, soft texture and sweet, slightly smoky flavour. Celeriac is a large, round, knobbly corm, related to celery. It has a similar flavour, but has a soft, creamy texture when cooked and a nutty one when raw or blanched. Once peeled, both vegetables need to be put immediately into acidulated water (with a little lemon juice added) to prevent browning.

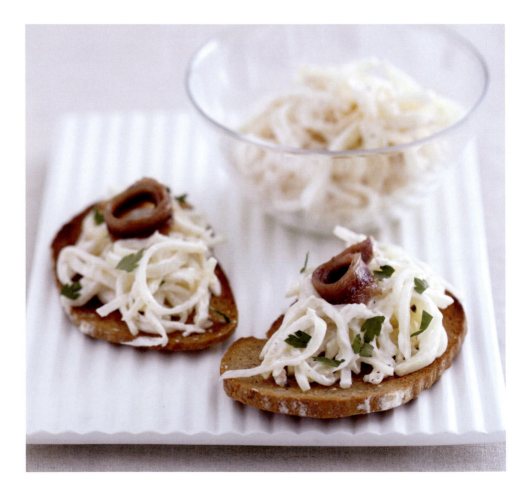

LUNCH ONLY   Remoulade toasts

People don't often think of eating Jerusalem artichokes raw, but they are delicious. You can make this with just one of the vegetables if you prefer. Blanch them as soon as you grate them or they will discolour. Serve as a light lunch or, without the toast, as an accompaniment to grilled oily fish for an evening meal.

Makes 4 portions

1 tbsp lemon juice
225g Jerusalem artichokes
½ small celeriac (about 225g)
2tbsp mayonnaise
2 tbsp natural yoghurt
1 tsp grated horseradish (fresh or from a jar)
1 tsp white balsamic
Freshly ground black pepper
8 slices rye bread
2 tbsp olive oil
A little chopped fresh parsley
50g can anchovy fillets, drained

1. Bring a pan of water to the boil and add the lemon juice. Peel the artichokes and celeriac and cut into thin matchsticks with a knife, or using a shredder attachment for a food processor. Drop the shredded vegetables immediately into the boiling acidulated water and blanch for 20 seconds. Drain, rinse with cold water, and drain again. Pat dry on kitchen paper.
2. Mix the mayonnaise, yoghurt, horseradish, and balsamic condiment together and season with pepper. Mix in the shredded vegetables. Chill until ready to serve.
3. Brush the bread all over with olive oil. Toast on both sides until golden. Leave to cool. Pile the remoulade on the toasts. Top each with a sprinkling of parsley and a curled anchovy fillet.

What to look for
• Choose clean specimens with the fewest knobbles and gnarls so they're easier to prepare.
• Both vegetables should feel heavy for their size.
• For Jerusalem artichokes, two pieces of joined tuber should snap apart easily.
• Avoid any that have soft brown patches.

Ways to cook or serve
• Salad
• Purée
• Gratin (in cheese sauce)
• Mash
• Soup
• Roast
• Griddle (celeriac)
• Stew or casserole

Simple ways to flavour
• Add nutmeg, crème fraîche, and a small knob of butter to a purée.
• Mash, purée, or roast and serve with game, red meats, or oily fish.
• Scatter fragrant herbs such as rosemary, sage, or thyme over when roasting.
• Toss toasted sesame seeds and a splash of toasted sesame oil in after roasting, or sprinkle over mash.

Avocados

This extremely nutritious fruit, which has the highest protein and oil content of all, has a wonderful creamy texture with pale-green flesh when ripe. There are two main varieties available: the rough-skinned, ovoid Hass, which turns black when ripe, and the large, shiny-green, pear-shaped Fuerte. Avocados are most often served raw, but can be cooked. If overcooked, however, they tend to become bitter, so care should be taken if preparing them this way. All avocados ripen off the tree, but if you buy them when completely hard they may never become fully ripe and be fibrous inside. To speed up the ripening process, place in a bag with a banana or apple, which give off a gas that speeds up this process.

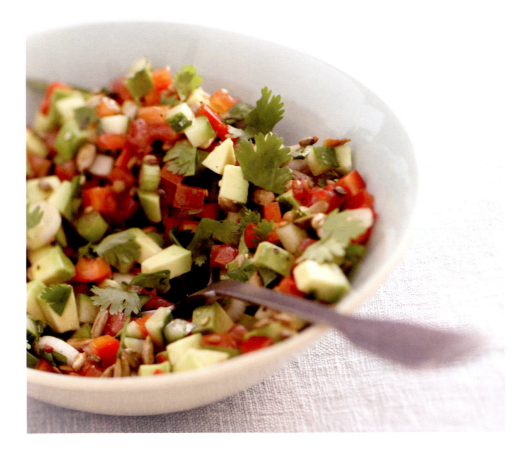

Avocado salsa

This makes a delicious light supper on its own. Alternatively, serve it in smaller quantities to accompany any spiced grilled fish, chicken, or meat in the evening, or with a spiced rice dish at lunchtime.

Makes 4 portions

2 large just-ripe avocados
4 spring onions, chopped
1 red pepper, halved, deseeded, and chopped
2 tomatoes, deseeded and chopped
1 fresh fat red chilli, deseeded and thinly sliced
¼ cucumber, chopped
30g sunflower seeds or seed mix
2 tbsp lime juice
2 tbsp olive oil
Freshly ground black pepper
2 tbsp roughly chopped fresh coriander, plus a few
    extra torn leaves

1. Halve the avocados, remove the stones, peel off the flesh, and cut the flesh into small dice.
2. Place in a bowl. Add all the remaining ingredients and toss gently until well-combined. Take care not to crush the avocado flesh.
3. Pile into a serving dish, scatter a few torn coriander leaves over the top, and chill until ready to serve.

Lunch only
Serve with a spiced rice dish such as Rice pilau with mushrooms and hazelnuts (p.148).

Complex carbohydrates

What to look for
• To check if an avocado is ripe (apart from Hass turning black), they should give gently when squeezed in the palm of your hand.
• Avoid any avocados with soft, bruised patches – they will be blackened inside.

Ways to cook or serve
• Salad
• Dips (like guacamole)
• Mousse
• Soup
• Salsa
• Grill
• Bake

Simple ways to flavour
• Crushed with lime juice for traditional guacamole or, for more flavour, add some chopped fresh chilli or dried chilli flakes, diced cucumber, and tomato and spike with Worcestershire sauce.
• Mash with a little lemon juice and beat with olive oil – a splash at a time – for a mayonnaise-like emulsion. Season and serve with seafood, chicken, or a salad.
• Fill the cavity (made by the stone) with French dressing, or prawns with Marie Rose sauce (mayonnaise and crème fraîche mixed together and flavoured with tomato purée and a few drops of Tabasco and Worcestershire sauce), or cottage cheese and chopped walnuts and snipped chives with a squeeze of lemon.

Bean sprouts and raw sprouted seeds

Sprouted beans, peas, and seeds have a lovely crunch and add texture, flavour, and colour to salads, sandwiches, wraps, and stir-fries. They are readily available, but can be grown at home very easily: Soak enough mung beans to cover the base of a plastic or glass container in an even layer in a bowl of tepid water for 12 hours. Drain, rinse well, and spread out evenly in the container. Cover with the container lid and place away from direct sunlight. Rinse twice a day for five to six days by gently pouring water over the beans, then draining off the water. When sprouted to the desired length, wash the sprouts well before use to remove the green husks.

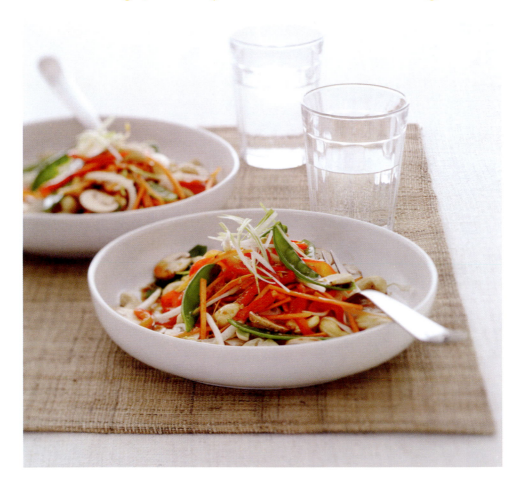

Bean sprout, roasted red pepper, and cashew nut salad

If buying ready-sprouted beans, choose ones that look and smell fresh and are not discolouring (if they are, they will soon start fermenting). You can also make this dish with raw red peppers if you are short of time.

Makes 4 portions

2 red peppers
115g mangetout
4 spring onions
1 large carrot, cut in thin matchsticks
115g fresh bean sprouts
115g raw cashew nuts
3 tbsp soy sauce
1 garlic clove, crushed
2 tbsp sunflower oil
1 tbsp white balsamic

1. Preheat the grill and roast the peppers for about 15 minutes, turning once or twice until the skin is blackened all over. Alternatively, turn on forks over a gas flame. Place in a plastic bag and leave to cool.
2. Meanwhile, steam the mangetout for 1–2 minutes. Drain, rinse with cold water, drain again, and place in a large bowl. Trim the spring onions, cut into 5cm lengths, and then into fine shreds. Reserve a quarter of the spring onions for garnishing and put the rest in the bowl with the mangetout.
3. Scrape off the blackened skins from the cooled peppers, then cut them in halves, remove the stalks and seeds, rinse, dry on kitchen paper, then cut into thin strips. Add to the bowl along with the carrot, bean sprouts, and cashew nuts.
4. Whisk the soy sauce with the garlic, sunflower oil, and balsamic condiment. Pour over the salad and toss gently until well combined. Chill until ready to serve.
5. Pile into salad bowls and serve cold, garnished with the reserved spring onion shreds.

Lunch only
Substitute udon noodles for the mangetout. Cook 3 bundles (250g) of noodles according to packet directions. Drain, rinse with cold water, and drain again. Place in the large bowl (step 2) and add the other ingredients.

Complex carbohydrates

What to look for
•Mung bean sprouts: good raw or lightly cooked in Asian dishes
•Radish sprouts: a lovely peppery flavour for salads and in wraps
•Pea sprouts (not to be confused with pea shoots, the tips of pea plants, sold as salad leaves)
•Mustard and/or cress, sold in small boxes. Can be grown at home, but on blotting paper or wet kitchen paper in a shallow dish. Look for red mustard, too.
•Alfalfa sprouts, from seeds
•Lentil sprouts
•Aduki bean sprouts

Ways to cook or serve
•Salad
•Stir-fry
•Sandwich
•Wrap or pancake
•Garnish

Simple ways to flavour
•With Asian flavours like fresh ginger, soy sauce, black bean or oyster sauce, and five-spice in stir-fries with vegetables and/or chicken, pork, beef, or seafood
•With a dressing of sunflower oil, soy sauce, garlic, and white balsamic condiment
•Hard boiled or scrambled egg with cress, mustard and cress, or radish sprouts in a sandwich
•With bulgur wheat, couscous, or cooked brown or red rice, chilli, cumin, chopped pimientos, sun-kissed tomatoes, grated courgettes and raw peas, topped with a spoonful of thick yoghurt

Celery and fennel

These both have crisp, juicy stalks with distinctive flavours. Fennel – often known as Florence fennel – is short and squat (don't confuse it with wild fennel, which is a herb with a similar aniseed flavour), while celery is long and thin. Both can be eaten raw or cooked on their own or as flavouring to many other dishes. Celery leaves and the soft, dark-green fronds of fennel can both be used for garnishing finished dishes. Fennel seeds are one of the oldest spices, long used to aid digestion and ease colic, but they also taste delicious. Celery seeds are tiny and an excellent addition to many dishes, imparting a delicate celery flavour and slight crunch.

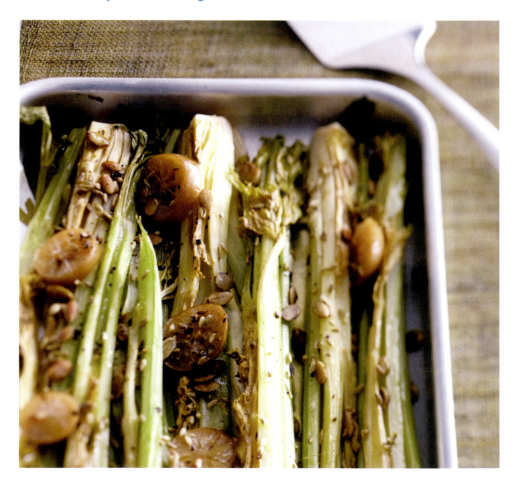

Roasted celery hearts or fennel with preserved lemon

This is a glorious side dish to serve with roasted meat, chicken, or chunky fish such as monkfish or cod loin, and accompanied by some couscous for lunch or quinoa for supper. The preserved lemons add a subtle citrusy flavour. You can turn it into a quick meal by adding some cubes of halloumi cheese for the last 5 minutes of cooking time.

Makes 4 portions

2 large or 4 small fennel bulbs or celery hearts (or half and half)
2 preserved lemons, sliced
4 tbsp olive oil
1 tsp fennel or celery seeds
2 tbsp pumpkin seeds
Freshly ground black pepper
A few grains coarse sea salt (optional)

1. Preheat the oven to 190°C (Gas 5). Trim the fennel or celery and cut each piece into quarters. Place in a roasting tin with the preserved lemon slices. Drizzle with the olive oil and toss well.
2. Scatter the seeds over and season with black pepper. Cover with foil and roast in the oven for 35 minutes. Remove the foil, turn the vegetables over gently, and roast for a further 10 minutes until golden.
3. Loosen the vegetables with a fish slice, transfer to a warm serving dish, season with a few grains of coarse sea salt, if you like, and serve hot.

Complex carbohydrates

What to look for
•There are two types of celery: white and green. They are both the same plant, but white celery is grown in the dark to give it a paler colour and yellowy green leaves. Green celery has a stronger flavour; white is more tender and is best for braising.
•Choose either with clean stalks and bright, fresh-looking leaves. Avoid if the stalks are browning or feel limp.

Ways to cook or serve
•Salad
•Braise
•Stir-fry
•Soup
•Roast
•Stew and casserole

Simple ways to flavour
•A stalk or two with walnuts and apple or a piece of cheese for a snack
•Braised and coated with cheese sauce, or make into a soup flavoured with blue or yellow hard cheese
•Chopped and cooked with any seafood, or raw in salad
•Roasted with any citrus zest (or try preserved lemons, left) or in salad with citrusy-flavoured mayonnaise
•The seeds sprinkled in salads, mixed with soft white cheese and with seafood

Cucumber and radishes
Although radishes are technically a root vegetable, and cucumber is a member of the squash family, they are both quintessential salad vegetables along with tomatoes and lettuce, and add great texture, colour, and flavour to dishes. However, they can also be cooked – radishes can be used instead of turnips in soups and stews, for example – and small ridge cucumbers are commonly used for pickling. If you buy a cucumber covered in tight plastic, remove the plastic before storing it in the chiller box of the fridge, as it will keep much better. Twist off any leaves from radishes so that they stay crisp.

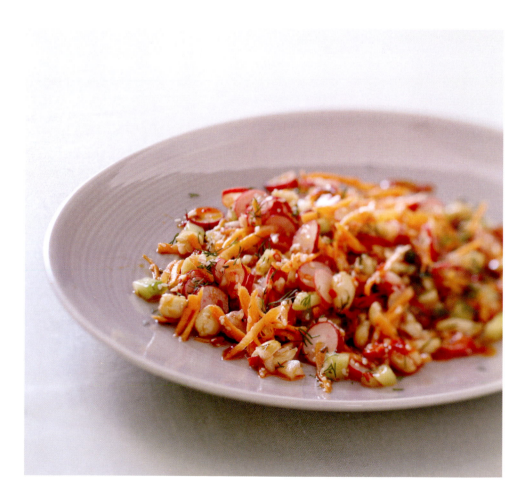

Cucumber and radish sambal salad

This mixture of fresh salad ingredients, peanuts, and seeds makes a delicious light meal topped with some natural yoghurt, if you like. It can also be served in smaller portions with or without the peanuts as an accompaniment to any spicy main course.

Makes 4 portions

½ cucumber
1 bunch of radishes, sliced
1 small onion, finely chopped
1 large carrot, coarsely grated
2 tbsp fresh chopped dill
115g roasted unsalted peanuts
2 tbsp sesame seeds
4 tbsp sunflower oil
2 tbsp apple juice
2 tbsp lime juice
2 tsp sambal oelek (chilli sauce)
Freshly ground black pepper

1. Cut the skin off the cucumber, cut in halves lengthways, scoop out the seeds with a teaspoon, then chop the flesh. Place in a large bowl.
2. Add the remaining prepared vegetables, dill, and nuts.
3. Whisk the remaining ingredients together and pour over the salad. Toss well and chill for at least 1 hour to allow the flavours to develop fully.

Lunch only
Serve with some wholemeal flatbreads (khobez).

What to look for
•Cucumbers: there are two types – the short ridge or outdoor variety, and the smooth, long European, or indoor, cucumber.
•Ridge cucumbers have tougher skin and larger seeds.
•Radishes: there are several types, but the most common are the round red ones and the elongated pink and white French breakfast ones.

Ways to cook or serve
•Salad
•Stir-fry
•Soup
•Pickle (ridge cucumbers)
•Gratin (cucumber in cheese sauce)
•Stuff (cucumbers)
•Steam (radishes)
•Stew (radishes)

Simple ways to flavour
•Cucumber cut into matchsticks and added to a stir-fry of seafood and carrots, celery and onions flavoured with ginger and soy sauce
•Cucumber and radishes thinly sliced and simply dressed with white-wine vinegar and freshly ground black pepper
•Cucumber and radishes grated with carrot and dressed with natural yoghurt, a splash of white balsamic, and fresh chopped mint or dill
•Radishes steamed whole and coated in parsley sauce

Salad leaves

This group covers every variety of lettuce head and all the individual leaves you can buy or grow. Some are available all year round, so there is always variety. They each have differing textures and flavours, but all add interest to other dishes and all are interchangeable according to taste. For chicory, always cut a cone shape out of the base of the head, which removes the bitterness. For watercress, trim the very bases of the feathery stalks, as they tend to be quite bitter. If buying boxes of cress, water regularly to keep the growing peat moist. To revive wilting leaves, put in a plastic bag, blow into the bag, and seal. Leave in the fridge for several hours. Store all lettuces and leaves in the chiller box in the fridge.

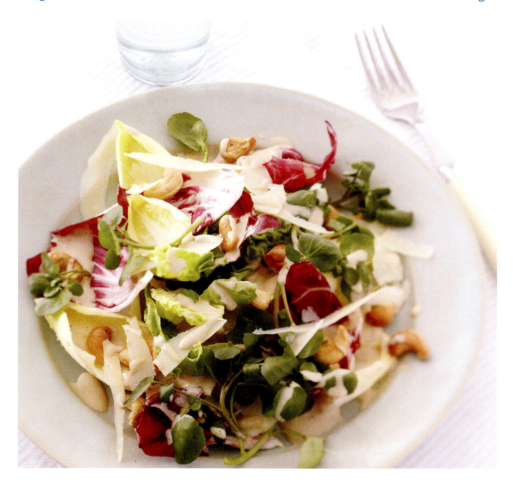

Mixed-leaf Caesar salad

Caesar salad is traditionally made just with romaine lettuce leaves, but this recipe has a whole selection for colour, flavour, and texture.

Makes 4 portions

1 small radicchio
1 little gem lettuce
1 head of chicory
½ bunch watercress (about 15g)
A handful of roasted, unsalted cashew nuts
For the dressing:
1 large egg
3 canned anchovy fillets
2 tsp Worcestershire sauce
3 tbsp sunflower oil
About ½ tsp lemon juice
Freshly ground black pepper
30g Parmesan or other Italian hard cheese, shaved with a potato peeler or on a mandolin

1. Trim the radicchio and little gem lettuce and separate into leaves. Tear into bite-sized pieces. Place in a large bowl. Cut a cone shape out of the base of the chicory (to remove the bitterness), cut the head into chunks and separate the leaves. Add to the bowl. Trim any thick stalks off the watercress and separate the sprigs into smaller ones. Add to the bowl with the nuts.
2. Boil the egg in water for just 1½ minutes. Drain and place immediately in cold water. When cool, crack the egg over a blender goblet or food processor and scoop the egg into it. Add the anchovies, Worcestershire sauce, and oil. Blend until thick and creamy, then sharpen to taste with lemon juice. Season with a good grinding of black pepper.
3. Spoon the dressing over and toss lightly. Pile into individual salad bowls, add the cheese shavings, and serve straight away.

Lunch only
Serve with garlic croutons.
2 thick slices cut from a large wholemeal loaf
2 tbsp milk
1 large garlic clove, crushed
Freshly ground black pepper
Preheat the oven to 220°C (Gas 7). Cut the bread into cubes. Toss in the milk and the crushed garlic. Spread on baking parchment on a baking sheet and bake for 10–12 minutes, or until crisp and golden. Remove from the oven. Add with the nuts in step 1.

Complex carbohydrates

What to look for
•Choose fresh-looking leaves. Avoid if wilting, bruised, or the white stalks are going brown.

Ways to cook or serve
•Lightly dressed
•Rocket or watercress piled on hot, freshly cooked pizza
•Braise (wedges or hearts)
•Soup
•Stir-fry
•Garnish
•Sandwich filling
•Large flat leaves for wraps, boat-shaped ones as receptacles

Simple ways to flavour
•French dressing: put a small spoonful of Dijon mustard in a screw-topped jar. Add 1 part white balsamic, 1 part white- or red-wine vinegar and 5–6 parts olive oil. Add some seasoning and shake vigorously. Add chopped fresh or a pinch of dried herbs, too, if you like.
•Flavoured vinegar, such as raspberry ,or flavoured oil, like chilli, truffle, or garlic, or garlic and herb cheese, thinned with a dash of olive oil and some milk adds extra depth. Finely grated orange zest and juice added to the oil with a splash of balsamic adds extra zing, too
•Shredded lettuce wedges or hearts stewed in a knob of butter with peas, chopped spring onions, and mint as a side dish

Tomatoes

There are hundreds of varieties of tomatoes in different shapes and sizes, and in colours from green (even when ripe) or cream, through yellow, orange, and red, right up to a deep rusty-black. Tomatoes are technically a fruit, but are served as a vegetable and are great raw or cooked. They are one of the most versatile ingredients, forming the basis of many dishes, and blend with everything from meat to fish and bread to rice. Storing in the fridge impairs their flavour – they should be kept in a fruit bowl or basket like apples.

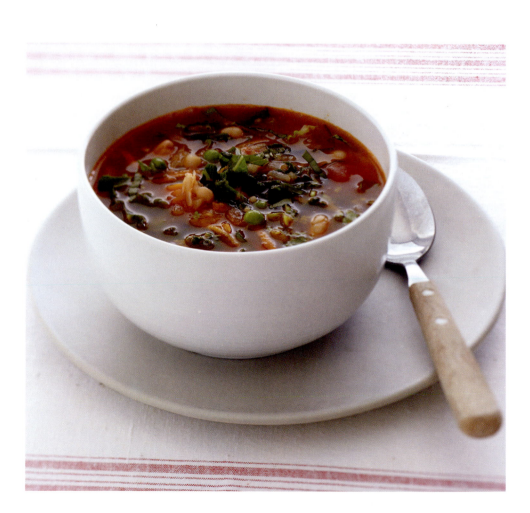

Minestrone soup

This tomato-based soup is a wonderful nutritious meal in a bowl. You can use swede instead of turnip, or ring the changes by adding finely chopped peppers or grated courgettes instead. If serving for lunch, you could add a handful of crushed wholewheat spaghetti with the rest of the ingredients.

Makes 4–6 portions

4 large, ripe tomatoes
1 onion, chopped
2 tbsp olive oil
1 carrot, grated
1 small turnip, grated
¼ small cabbage or 1 small head spring greens (about 115g),
    finely shredded, discarding any thick stump
55g frozen peas
2 tbsp tomato purée
410g can haricot beans in water, drained
    (or 240g cooked [115g raw weight] beans)
1.2 litres strong vegetable stock
1 tsp anchovy paste (optional)
1 bay leaf
Freshly ground black pepper
2 tbsp chopped fresh basil
Parmesan or other Italian hard cheese, or Cheddar cheese,
    grated (optional)

1. Put the tomatoes in a bowl. Cover with boiling water, leave to stand for 30 seconds, then lift out the tomatoes. Peel off the skins and chop the flesh. Put to one side.
2. Fry the onion in the oil in a large pan for 1 minute, stirring. Add the tomatoes and all the remaining ingredients except the basil.
3. Bring to the boil, reduce the heat, part-cover, and simmer gently for 10 minutes, or until the vegetables are really tender. Discard the bay leaf. Add the basil. Taste and re-season, if necessary.
4. Ladle into soup bowls and serve sprinkled liberally with cheese, if using.

Lunch only
Serve with wholegrain bread.

Complex carbohydrates

What to look for
•Best to buy on the vine, when possible, for optimum flavour.
•Cherry: baby round ones to eat whole or halved in salads
•Plum: great flavour for cooking with (these are the ones sold in cans). Baby plums are great with pasta, rice, and couscous.
•Standard: all-purpose round tomatoes
•Beefsteak: extra-large tomatoes for salads, sauces, sandwiches, or stuffing
•Canned whole or chopped, passata (sieved tomatoes), sun-dried, sun-kissed (semi-dried) and concentrated tomato purée

Ways to cook or serve
•Raw in salads and snacks
•Grill
•Sauté
•Stew
•Soup
•Juice
•Sauce
•Pizza topping

Simple ways to flavour
• Sauté cherry tomatoes on the vine in a little olive oil, carefully turning once. Add balsamic vinegar and allow to bubble. Serve with the juices on top.
•Herbs (chopped, fresh): basil, rosemary, thyme, chives, mint, coriander, and parsley
•Add orange zest and juice to bring out the fruitiness of tomato soup.
•Any protein

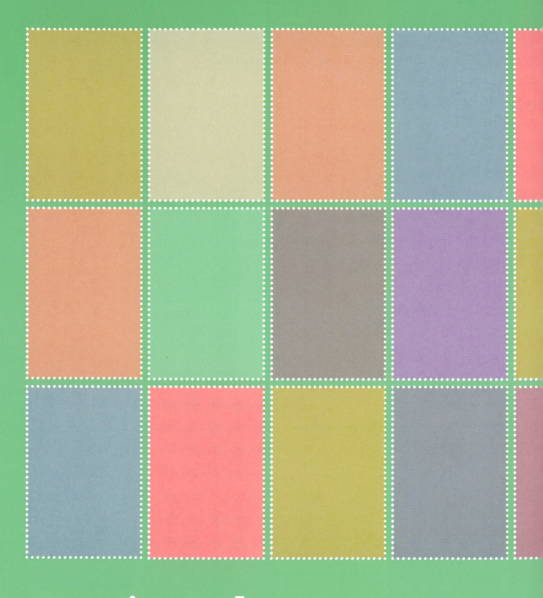

Section three

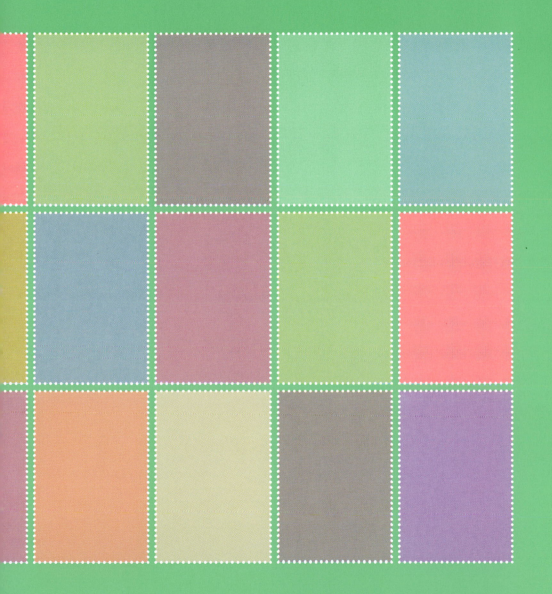

Food planners

Introduction

Having looked at how to eat in Section one, and at the typical foods you might choose to eat in Section two, we'll now see how to make my plan work for you and how to adapt it to your own lifestyle.

Depending on our age and circumstances, how we live our lives can differ enormously. With this in mind, I have put together ten diverse case studies of people at various ages and stages. After learning a little about their current circumstances, and their occasionally poor food choices, we'll look at how they can each change their eating habits for the better and what they might eat instead. I have devised a food planner for each case study that covers three separate days – either two weekdays (one more rushed than the other) and one day at the weekend when there is usually a little more time to think about food, or a whole weekend and one weekday. The focus will be on eating the food groups together and at frequent regular intervals. These food planners will show you how easy it can be to create a simple and nutritious menu that fits into your lifestyle; just work out which case study you most identify with – or children that you need to cater for – and use the food planner as a blueprint that you can adapt and vary by referring to the meal and snack suggestions and recipes in Section two.

When I work with clients on a one-to-one basis, they often tell me that they don't have time to cook, or that they work too hard to have time to break off from what they are doing to eat a snack mid-morning. I have no doubt that time is an issue for all of us, but it is important to understand that eating regularly is essential, and it doesn't have to be at all complicated. No cooking is required to make an instant snack if that's what you require – it's simply a question of putting together a couple of different foods from the fridge, or buying them in a food store on your morning commute, if you work in an office. When it comes to cooking, I know that when I look at a recipe I sometimes find myself thinking that it might look delicious, but will I actually find the time to make it? I don't have the time to buy the ingredients, let alone actually cook... but then I remind myself that I do have to buy food to eat anyway, and none of the ingredients in the recipe look unusual. All it really means is that I have to add a couple of extra ingredients to my shopping basket when I'm at the grocery store. When I cook the recipe, it is always worthwhile and far quicker and easier than I imagined. I also make a point of preparing more than I need for that meal so that I have a couple of extra portions to enjoy over the following day or two – creating a couple of instant meals in the process, and saving myself more time than I initially factored in.

There is one important point to make at this juncture: eating well does take a little time, thought, and effort. However, it doesn't have to take much thought, as the *How Not To Get Fat* principles will become second nature to you after a day or two, and neither does it take much time or effort once you become familiar with your new routine.

After an initial consultation with clients, I ask them not to start their new approach to eating the very next day, but to do something else for themselves by way of preparation. I ask them to carry on making the same food choices for one more day, but make a note of what they might eat instead if they were on my plan. For example, clients who come to me for advice on increasing their energy levels might always buy a low-fat muffin and a skinny cappuccino for breakfast on their way to work. They might see that at the same café they can choose a decaffeinated coffee and a croissant with ham instead. They may also understand that had they eaten something at home, however small it was, within an hour of getting up, their hunger would be diminished and their energy levels increased. Throughout the day they will learn what they might have eaten, and by the following day they usually feel quite confident about making these beneficial changes. You may wish to try this approach as well: write down what you eat for a day or two and think about what you might have eaten instead of, or in addition to, your usual choices so that you combine the different food groups (pp.16–17) and eat at regular intervals.

Carol and Tim

Carol lives with her husband, Tim, and they have three grown-up children. The eldest, Mark, 34, lives with his wife, Emma, and their two children. Carol and Tim have a daughter, Laura, 26, who works in London, and their youngest, Greg, is 20 years old and at university. Carol used to be a full-time homemaker, but now that the children have left home she spends her time enjoying hobbies. Tim still works five days a week, leaving home before 8am and returning by 7pm. Carol and Tim have a busy social life and often have friends over to dinner. One weekend a month Carol and Tim visit Greg at university, when Carol takes the opportunity to fill Greg's fridge-freezer with some of her home-cooked meals.

Both Carol and Tim have gained weight as they have got older, but since the children left home Carol has been more active and plays golf twice a week when the weather allows, and Tim plays golf at the weekends. Carol tries to follow a low-calorie diet, but feels it isn't possible when playing golf or socializing, so she often diets for a few days here and there and relies on her golf to burn off the calories. She eats fruit for breakfast and sometimes has a bowl of porridge as well, especially if she is playing golf. Carol often has just soup for lunch, as she prefers to eat the proper meal she makes for herself and Tim in the evening – usually chicken with vegetables, and a potato side dish for Tim as well. When the couple entertains or eats out, Carol eats what she wants and then tries to eat carefully the rest of the week. Her chosen drink is low-calorie tonic with vodka, as it contains the least calories. Tim relies upon Carol to plan what they eat, as she does most of the shopping, and instinctively chooses his favourite foods for lunch when he's at work.

Carol eats too little at times; instead she should aim for a consistent intake of food, and as she has time at home during the day she is well-placed to make sure that she has enough food in the house for snacks as well as main meals. Carol may shy away from foods such as nuts and seeds, as she thinks they might be 'fattening', but it is important that she understands the concept of combining foods and doesn't see food simply for its calorie content. Tim needs to be more aware of his food choices, and should make sure he is comfortable with the different snacks and meals he can choose. Carol can also ensure that he has the right sorts of foods for snacks in the office, perhaps buying nut butter, fresh nuts, and seeds for him to leave in his desk.

FOOD PLANNER FOR CAROL AND TIM

WEEKEND DAY 1

Breakfast

Carol: cornflakes with toasted almonds and sliced apple
Tim: toast with smoked salmon and a glass of juice
Both have a decaffienated coffee

Mid-morning snack

Fresh fruit and mixed nuts while shopping

Lunch

Warm chicken liver salad (p.35) with wholegrain bread

Afternoon snack

Carol: natural yoghurt and fruit salad topped with seeds
Tim: wholemeal pitta bread and houmous

Dinner

Carol and Tim have friends for dinner
With pre-dinner drinks: a selection of mixed raw nuts, olives, and houmous with crudités
Starter: Griddled asparagus with soft-boiled eggs (p.157)
Carol serves toasted English muffins with the asparagus to her guests, but she and Tim don't eat them.
Main course: Grilled pork chops with mustard sauce with chive mash (p.57).
Carol makes potato and celeriac mash to accompany the pork chops, and she and Tim choose the celeriac mash.
Final course: cheese platter, fruit salad with meringues
Carol and Tim enjoy two small glasses of red wine and have cheese instead of the sweet dessert.

WEEKEND DAY 2

Breakfast

Porridge with roasted hazelnuts and sliced peach and green tea or decaffeinated coffee

....

Mid-morning snack

Last night's leftover houmous with crudités

....

Lunch

Roast beef, a couple of roast potatoes, half a Yorkshire pudding, and plenty of vegetables

....

Afternoon snack

Carol and Tim don't have a snack, as they didn't finish lunch until 3pm.

....

Dinner

Early-evening supper of leftovers from last night's dinner party and a large salad scattered with mixed seeds

....

WEEKDAY

Breakfast

Carol and Tim both have porridge with chopped banana and toasted almonds and a decaffeinated coffee each.

Snack

Carol: As she is playing golf today, Carol packs some dried apricots and a palmful of Brazil nuts for the car journey.
Tim: some dried apricots and a palmful of Brazil nuts at his desk

Lunch

Carol: chicken Caesar salad in the clubhouse
Tim: chicken salad sandwich from a local café

Afternoon snack

Carol: houmous with wholemeal pitta bread
Tim: a banana and some more Brazil nuts

Dinner

Home-made beef burgers and Curried spring greens with Cashew Nuts (p.161)

Carol makes and freezes extra burgers to give her son, Greg, when she and Tim drive over visit him at university at the weekend.

Chris is in his late 20s and is an IT consultant for a music company. He has a flat-share and travels to work every day. He isn't a confident cook, but he can make pasta and other very basic recipes. He would like to cook more, but isn't at home that much. He leaves home at 7.30am, gets breakfast on the way to work, and rarely returns home before 9pm. Chris has a passion for music and goes to gigs whenever he can get tickets from the office, which is usually a couple of times a week. He doesn't worry about his weight and his friends often say that he can eat what he likes without putting on any weight. He is aware of the concept of 'eating well', but doesn't like the idea of ever having to diet or restrict what foods he eats as his girlfriends do.

Chris usually buys a plain croissant and a café latte on his journey into work. He drinks coffee or water at the office to keep him going if he gets tired and hungry, as he doesn't get time to eat until lunch, which is a sandwich or wrap from the cafeteria. In the afternoon he drinks more coffee and has some sweet biscuits and a chocolate bar. If he is going out straight from work, Chris eats a sandwich and a cola drink as he leaves the office. If he stays out late, he often gets a pizza or kebab on the way home. On the nights that he is home he will eat a ready-made meal or make some pasta with a sauce and vegetables.

This plan will suit Chris well, as he doesn't have to restrict himself and resist foods in the same way that he has seen his girlfriends do. Chris will need to make sure that he has stocks of easy-to-cook proteins such as eggs, canned fish, and canned beans in his store-cupboard so that he can easily add protein to his late-night snacks.

FOOD PLANNER FOR CHRIS

WEEKDAY 1

Pre-breakfast snack

An apple and some almonds at 7am

Breakfast

On the way to work Chris buys breakfast, plus some food for a mid-morning snack. He can still have his usual croissant and coffee, but he should choose a ham croissant and a decaffeinated café latte.

Mid-morning snack

A small bottle of apple juice and an oat and seed bar (from his breakfast café) with a palmful of walnuts

Lunch

Chicken salad sandwich from the cafeteria

Afternoon snack

A banana and some mixed nuts

Late afternoon snack

Before leaving work to meet friends, Chris has a wholemeal roll with beef, lettuce, and tomato, bought from the caféteria at lunchtime.

Dinner

Arriving home at 10pm, Chris eats 2 slices of cheese with the Cucumber and radish sambal salad (p.189) that he made the night before (and prepared extra portions).

WEEKEND DAY 1

Breakfast
Scrambled eggs with bacon and a slice of brown toast

Mid-morning snack
A bowl of wholegrain cereal with flaked almonds

Lunch
Chris meets some friends for lunch in a restaurant and has spaghetti with bolognaise sauce and a couple of bottles of beer.

Afternoon snack
At the cinema with his friends, Chris has a small bag of mixed nuts, shares a small tub of salted popcorn, and drinks a bottle of sparkling water.

Dinner
Chris cooks a beef and vegetable stir-fry (p.47) with extra steamed vegetables before meeting friends for drinks at the pub.
Coming home later in the evening, he eats some leftovers from dinner if he is hungry again and intends to stay up for a couple of hours.

WEEKEND DAY 2

Breakfast
Cooked English breakfast and decaffeinated coffee at a local café

Mid-morning snack
An apple and a palmful of Brazil nuts

Lunch
Pasta bake (p.140) with a green salad

Afternoon snack
Chris finishes off the leftovers of the pasta bake from lunch.

Dinner
Chris has an Indian takeaway with his flatmates: tandoori chicken and mixed vegetable curry. He avoids the white rice and naan breads, and enjoys 2 poppadoms instead.

Claire is in her early 30s, lives alone in her own flat, and works long

hours in marketing. Claire considers herself to be healthy and well-informed about food and health. She finds time to go to the gym twice a week, and also swims once a week. If she gains a little weight over Christmas, say, she increases her exercise to compensate and is a little more careful about what she eats until she is back to her usual size 10 again. Claire is aware that her mother is overweight and is adamant that she won't allow herself to put on weight in the same way. However, she does tend to get taken in by quick-fix diets that she reads about in magazines, often following them for a few days or a couple of weeks before giving up. Claire enjoys cooking and eating her own food, but is often hungry and feels quite tired at the end of each working day, as she uses willpower to control her food intake.

Claire eats muesli for breakfast with skimmed milk and a cup of green tea. At the office she has a bottle of water on her desk and drinks it throughout the day. She eats dried fruit if she is hungry. Claire brings her lunch in from home, which is often a large salad with canned tuna or salmon. Before going to the gym or swimming pool after work, Claire will eat a banana, but because she usually gets home quite late after this exercise she tends to have home-made soup or put a premium ready-made meal in the microwave.

Claire can become immune to the celebrity diets she reads about by learning how to eat, not how to diet. She must ensure that she always eats breakfast and also learn not to fear hunger; instead of living with hungry feelings, she can respond to her hunger by eating complex carbohydrates and protein together.

FOOD PLANNER FOR CLAIRE

WEEKEND

Breakfast
Poached eggs on wholegrain toast and a
decaffeinated cappuccino

Mid-morning snack
Goats cheese and sliced cucumber on half of
a multi-seed bagel

Lunch
Curried quinoa and vegetable pilaf (p.84) and a glass of
white wine. Claire makes an extra portion of the pilaf for
lunch at work the next day.

Afternoon snack
Avocado salsa (p.183) on 2 oatcakes

Dinner
Poached salmon (p.102) with Stir-fried beans and
mangetout (p.167), making an extra portion to store in
the fridge to eat in the next day or so.

WEEKDAY 1

Breakfast

Nut-rich muesli with skimmed milk and a cup of green tea.
Claire also takes a portion of home-made Minestrone soup (p.193) out of the freezer and leaves it in the fridge at home to defrost.

Mid-morning snack

Salmon paste (made at home before work with some of last night's leftover poached salmon mixed with a little mayonnaise and a drizzle of lemon juice) on 2 oatcakes

Lunch

Cold Curried quinoa and vegetable pilaf (left over from the weekend) and sparkling water

Afternoon snack

Dried apricots, mixed nuts and peppermint tea

Late afternoon snack

Before leaving the office to swim, Claire eats another oatcake with some more home-made salmon paste.

Dinner

Thawed, reheated soup from the freezer, followed by the rest of last night's leftover cold poached salmon with cold Stir-fried beans and mangetout

WEEKDAY 2

Breakfast

Porridge with a heaped tablespoon of vanilla mixed nuts (p.78) and a sliced banana

Mid-morning snack

2 oatcakes spread with houmous

Lunch

Claire has lunch with a client. She orders Salade Niçoise and one glass of red wine.

Afternoon snack

A small tub of natural yoghurt with a small packet of trail mix (mixed dried fruit and nuts) stirred into it

Dinner

Grilled chicken breast (p.35) and Roasted celery hearts with preserved lemon (p.187)

Emma is in her mid-30s and lives with her husband, Mark. They have two children, five-year-old Jack and two-year-old Daisy. Emma works part time from 9.15am to 5pm three days a week. This late start at work gives her enough time to drop Jack at school before taking Daisy on to nursery. On the days she works, Emma's mother collects both children and takes them back to their house to look after them until Emma gets home. Mark leaves the house at 8am and returns around 6.30pm. Emma enjoys cooking, but feels that she has no time to organise and prepare proper meals since the children were born. As well as cooking for the children, Emma does her best to make a meal for Mark in the evening, but often resorts to the most basic of meals. Emma lost weight for her wedding seven years ago, gained much of it back when she was pregnant with Jack, lost some of it again after the birth, and then regained more weight before Daisy was born. Emma is still heavier than she would like to be, but doesn't have the time or inclination to join a weight-loss group. She would prefer to exercise, but time always evaporates before she gets round to it and then she feels too tired to make the effort.

Typically, Emma eats low-calorie cereal on its own for breakfast, usually with a cup of tea, and on the days she works she has tea and fruit mid-morning and a sandwich for lunch. She doesn't usually eat again until the early evening, when she picks at what she is making for the children and finishes whatever they leave on their plates. By the time Mark gets home, Emma's appetite has diminished and she feels so tired that she makes whatever is quickest and easiest for dinner – often a ready-made meal cooked in the microwave.

Emma understands that her children have to be fed, but feels that she can manage without eating a balanced diet, which we know isn't the case and has led to her low levels of energy and weight fluctuations in the past. Emma has plenty to do every day and might feel that she doesn't have the energy to cook interesting meals, but if she eats in the way that I have planned for her, then her energy levels should rise.

FOOD PLANNER FOR EMMA

WEEKEND

Breakfast
Scrambled eggs with rye toast, grilled tomatoes, and a cup of tea

Mid-morning snack
Yoghurt, avocado, and cucumber dip (p.64) with wholemeal pitta bread
The children like to eat the dip with carrot sticks and Emma makes extra to take to work for snacks.

Lunch
Pasta bake (p.140) served with a Bean sprout, roasted red pepper, and cashew nut salad (p.185) for Mark and Emma, and puréed carrots for the children

Afternoon snack
Toast and peanut butter while making a batch of home-made soup (p.171, p.193) – some of which Emma freezes – and preparing home-made chicken burgers for dinner

Dinner
Chicken burgers (p.35) with mashed potato and peas for the children, and Stir-fried green beans and mangetout (p.167) for Emma and Mark

EMMA

WEEKDAY 1 (WORK DAY FOR EMMA)

Breakfast

Porridge with berries and flaked almonds (the children have the same)

Mid-morning snack

Some of yesterday's Yoghurt, avocado, and cucumber dip (p.64) on 2 oatcakes, with a few walnuts

Lunch

Store-bought tuna sandwich and an apple

Mid-afternoon snack

Store-bought houmous and 2 rye crackers

Late afternoon snack

A bowl of soup with half a can of chick-peas added to it while the children eat their dinner

Dinner

After the children are in bed, Emma quickly cooks some fish fillets (pp.114–15) and pre-cut vegetables.

Breakfast

Shredded wheat, half a banana, and some mixed vanilla nuts (p.78) before dropping off the children and going on to the gym

Mid-morning snack

Protein shake and an apple immediately after exercising

Lunch

Tomato and mozzarella salad followed by grilled tuna with spinach and polenta

Afternoon snack

Houmous with crudités
The children have the same when they come in from school. Emma roasts two chickens, serving some to the children with a little mashed potato and some green beans for their dinner. She puts one chicken aside to cool and store in the fridge to make an open chicken sandwich with vegetables and some flavoured oil for lunch the next day, with enough left over to add to some pasta for the children's supper and to make a chicken curry for Mark and herself in the evening.

Dinner

Cold roast chicken with a vegetable dish

EMMA

Greg is 20 and is in his second year at university. Having spent his first year on campus in a hall of residence, he is now sharing a house with three male students. Greg grew up with his mother, Carol, cooking all his food, and since he left home he has tried to cook from time to time although his repertoire is limited by ability and budget. He quite enjoys making his own food, but his housemates tend to rely on takeaways and instant snacks so there is always convenience or junk food in the house. Greg is relishing the freedom of being away from home, but as he doesn't have much money to spend on food he appreciates the occasional visits from his parents, who bring him some home-made food and take him out for a proper meal. Greg plays football a couple of times a week and enjoys the social life that university has to offer, although he often drinks more beer than he intends to. He and his housemates fend for themselves during the week, but try to eat dinner together once a week.

Greg usually eats cereal or toast for breakfast and then a ham or cheese roll mid-morning if there is a break in lectures; if not, he will make do with a can of cola. Often he makes it through to lunch and then eats two sandwiches with another can of cola. Before playing football he has a sandwich and then a few drinks afterwards before getting home late and eating a large bowl of cereal. On the nights when he or his housemates eat together, they usually cook a large quantity of pasta and add a store-bought sauce.

Because Greg is a student, he has to manage his budget quite carefully. Eating well doesn't mean spending more, however, as he can still use inexpensive complex carbohydrates such as pasta and add protein in the form of beans or cheese. The energy these sorts of foods create is broken down more slowly by the body, leaving Greg feeling fuller for longer so that he doesn't have to reach for junk food and soft drinks.

FOOD PLANNER FOR GREG

WEEKDAY 1

Breakfast
Cereal sprinkled with pumpkin seeds, or toast with sugar-free peanut butter

Mid-morning snack
A cheese roll and a smoothie, bought on the way to lectures

Lunch
A baked potato with beans and salad and a small bottle of sparkling water, bought from the caféteria on campus

Mid-afternoon snack
An apple, a banana, and a small pack of unsalted peanuts

Dinner
Omelette (p.42) made with green beans, ham, and peppers, saving a quarter of the omelette for breakfast the next morning

Breakfast

2 slices of toast with leftover omelette and a cup of tea

Mid-morning snack

A bowl of muesli with a few extra nuts added (Greg is studying at home)

Lunch

2 bowls of home-made Minestrone soup (p.193) with sliced ham and grated Cheddar cheese on top, and 2 slices of wholemeal bread

Afternoon snack

2 slices of wholemeal toast with peanut butter

Dinner

Chicken, shiitake mushroom, and pak-choi stir-fry (p.36) – but with spring greens instead of the pak choi and button mushrooms, as they are less expensive for Greg and his housemates. The housemates eat rice with their meal but Greg has extra vegetables instead.

Breakfast

Cereal with pumpkin seeds and sliced banana

Mid-morning snack

Wholemeal bread or a roll with sliced ham and tomato

Lunch

Greg meets his parents for lunch and has lamb shank with mashed potato and carrots. Afterwards he shares a chocolate mousse with his mother. His mother's food package includes home-made burgers, which he stores in the fridge.

Afternoon snack

2 slices of wholemeal toast with peanut butter

Dinner

2 home-made beef burgers with Crushed roasted carrots, chick-peas, and crumbled feta (p.163)

GREG

Kerry

Kerry is in her mid-30s and is a vegetarian. She has been dating John for some time, but usually sees him only at weekends. She is a full-time lawyer working for a large firm and often works long hours. She would like to lose some weight, but associates weight loss with exercise and, as she feels she has no free time to exercise, she prioritises work instead. She can't be bothered with proper food shops and finding interesting recipes to cook – it's difficult to find time to look for vegetarian recipes that appeal.

As a result, Kerry has let her diet slip and on a typical day she might skip breakfast and have a cup of coffee instead. She rarely eats until lunchtime, when she usually has either a cheese salad or pasta and salad from the caféteria at work, which is open from 7am to 10pm. Kerry has fluctuating energy levels through her long working day, and finds it hard to know what to eat at work as a vegetarian – she tends to eat the same thing most days. Kerry switches to tea in the afternoon, and she might have a piece of fruit or a couple of biscuits around 4pm. She will often pick up a ready-made meal on her way home to cook in the microwave. Kerry will only be able to eat well if it is very easy to plan and execute, and doesn't take up her precious free time.

Kerry works long hours and feels that she doesn't have time to eat. When we are stressed, adrenaline is released to supply short-term energy, but it also masks hunger pangs. Abstaining from eating is not the way to manage weight in the long term, so Kerry needs to eat even if she is only marginally hungry. This might mean having smaller portions, but she does need to eat every two and a half to three hours.

FOOD PLANNER FOR KERRY

WEEKDAY 1

Pre-breakfast snack
A couple of tablespoons of natural yoghurt with a few pumpkin seeds and a glass of grapefruit juice before leaving for work at 6.30am

Breakfast
A bowl of porridge bought from a café near work, to which Kerry adds a handful of pecans from a bag she keeps in her desk drawer

Mid-morning snack
An apple and a handful of the pecans

Lunch
A baked potato with beans and a salad from the office cafe

Afternoon snack
Shop-bought houmous with sliced carrots (store-bought or prepared at home the night before)

Early evening snack
Still working at the office at 7pm, Kerry has a bowl of vegetable soup with some grated cheese on top

Dinner
On getting home at 9pm Kerry makes a quick omelette (p.42) with red peppers

KERRY

Breakfast

Fruit salad with seeds and natural yoghurt. Kerry then catches a train to a meeting out of town and has a peppermint tea.

Mid-morning snack

An apple and some nuts from a bag in Kerry's briefcase as she travels

Lunch

Pasta with a tomato sauce in a café, but with 2 spoonfuls of mozzarella and pine nuts from the salad bar scattered on top of the dish

Afternoon snack

On the return journey, Kerry has a granola bar with a small palmful of nuts and a cup of tea from the snack bar onboard the train.

Dinner

Getting home at a decent hour, Kerry has time to make Tofu and sugar snap pea green curry (p.96).

Breakfast

Muesli with some vanilla-scented nuts (p.78)
Kerry then goes food shopping.

Mid-morning snack

John comes over for brunch and Kerry makes Quick eggs florentine (p.43).

Lunch

Kerry and John have a late lunch of Flatbread pizza with roasted pepper, beetroot and goats cheese (p.153).

Afternoon snack

A couple of slices of leftover Flatbread pizza

Dinner

Chick-pea and aubergine ragout without the pork (p.69)

KERRY

Margaret

Margaret is in her late 60s and was widowed five years ago. She used to cook every day, but now feels that it isn't worth cooking for just one person and only makes proper meals when her children and grandchildren stay with her. She usually snacks whenever she feels hungry, usually having some biscuits and a cup of coffee, which she also has when she plays bridge two mornings a week with her friends. When she shops, Margaret usually buys just a few fresh vegetables, some cooked meats, canned food, and a small loaf of white bread, as these foods are easy to store and won't spoil too quickly. She doesn't think it's worth buying too much fresh fruit and vegetables, as she worries she can't use them up quickly enough. She also often feels too full to eat fruit at the end of her meal, which is when she traditionally ate it. She feels she doesn't have much of an appetite anymore, but she doesn't have the same energy levels she used to enjoy.

On a typical day Margaret might eat cereal for breakfast, and then have a cup of tea and some sweet biscuits around 11am. For lunch she often has half a can of tomato soup and a piece of toast, and then a cup of tea and some more sweet biscuits in the afternoon. For dinner Margaret might eat cold sliced ham with some hot new potatoes.

Margaret has long been used to cooking for other people and it is hard to for her to be enthusiastic about cooking just for one. However, she simply needs to remember to cobble the right food groups together – so adding a slice of ham to her toast at lunch, or having cheese with crackers instead of sweet biscuits as a snack will make a significant difference to her energy levels and her interest in eating well. And rather than avoiding fruit altogether, she can enjoy it as part of a snack or breakfast.

FOOD PLANNER FOR MARGARET

WEEKDAY 1

Breakfast
Margaret can eat her usual cereal, but with a sliced banana and some toasted flaked almonds sprinkled on top, and enjoy a cup of tea.

Mid-morning snack
A slice of hard cheese with an apple

Lunch
Margaret might have her tomato soup and a slice of toast as usual, but with a slice of ham or shop-bought or home-made mackerel pâté spread on the toast.

Afternoon snack
2 oatcakes with cottage cheese

Dinner
Pan-roasted salmon (p.102) and capers with some frozen peas and fresh carrots

Breakfast

Cereal with flaked almonds and sliced apple, and
a cup of tea

Mid-morning snack

A pear and a slice of cheese

Lunch

Margaret makes a chicken casserole (p.34), as her
grandchildren have come to stay, and serves it with green
beans and mashed sweet potato. She makes an extra
portion to store in the fridge for lunch in a couple of days.

Afternoon snack

2 oatcakes with leftover mackerel pâté

Dinner

Margaret makes Spinach and cottage cheese frittata (p.45)
for herself and the grandchildren.

WEEKEND DAY 2

Breakfast
Margaret makes scrambled eggs and toast for herself and the grandchildren.

Mid-morning snack
As Margaret is out and about with her grandchildren, she buys a cereal and seed snack bar when she stops for a cup of tea.

Lunch
Margaret and the grandchildren have lunch in a pizza restaurant. Margaret has a chicken salad, while the children eat pizza.

Afternoon snack
Some dried apricots and almonds

Dinner
Toasted halloumi and pine nut salad (p.60)

Marie

has two teenage children, works full time since her divorce, and enjoys an active social life. She has gained and lost weight over the years since she was a teenager and has followed several diets in the past without long-term success. Typically, Marie has tried to follow a high-protein diet from time to time, but then craves carbohydrates, gives in, and eats lots of refined starchy carbohydrates until she can summon up the willpower to cut them out of her diet again.

Having reached her heaviest weight in the last two years, Marie recently embarked on a three-month plan of drinking meal-replacement shakes. She went from a size 20 to a 12 and was delighted with the results. She is eating meals again, but is worried about putting on weight once more. She tries to be very careful about what she eats, and is often hungry. Marie tends to have a low-calorie sweetened fruit yoghurt for breakfast when she gets to work, and a couple of fat-free biscuits before lunch if she is hungry. She drinks black coffee or tea without milk and plenty of water. Lunch is a packet of instant soup in a cup, and by the middle of the afternoon, when her willpower flags, she has another low-fat sweetened fruit yoghurt and some fresh fruit. Dinner at home is fish or a baked potato without butter or dressing (as Marie counts calories) with vegetables. If she eats out in the evening, she usually succumbs to something from the breadbasket, gets annoyed with herself, then decides to blow it all and order pasta or pizza, and tries to be extra 'good' the following day to compensate for her indulgence.

Marie is a classic dieter who lives with hunger and sees it as an almost normal way of life. By eating a combination of the food groups little and often, Marie will find that her hunger is greatly reduced. At times she may be tempted to skip snacks if she isn't hungry, but she should always eat something, however small it is, to keep her glucose levels consistent and avoid making poor food choices when she gets really hungry.

FOOD PLANNER FOR MARIE

WEEKDAY 1

Breakfast
A portion of bran flakes with sliced pear and sprinkled with flaked almonds
A cup of decaffeinated coffee

Mid-morning snack
Two rye crackers with cottage cheese and cucumber

Lunch
Marie can have her usual instant vegetable soup, but she should stir in a small can of mixed beans to eat with it.

Afternoon snack
Low-fat houmous with sliced carrots (prepared at home or bought ready-sliced)

Late afternoon snack
Marie has a small bag of unsalted nuts before she leaves work, as she is meeting friends for a drink.

Dinner
When she gets home around 9pm, Marie could eat some sliced chicken with a salad.

WEEKDAY 2

Breakfast

Two eggs with one slice of toasted rye bread
A glass of grapefruit juice

Mid-morning snack

2 slices of ham wrapped in lettuce on 2 oatcakes

Lunch

A salad made in the office kitchen with a pack of salad leaves, a few cherry tomatoes, an avocado, 1 can of tuna, and some walnuts

Afternoon snack

Fruit salad topped with mixed seeds

Dinner

Chicken, shiitake mushroom, and pak choi stir-fry (p.36)

WEEKEND

Breakfast

Porridge with pecans and a chopped banana

Mid-morning snack

A small portion of leftover stir-fried chicken from last night's meal

Lunch

Marie eats out and has goats cheese salad with a piece of wholegrain bread from the breadbasket, followed by grilled veal chop with spinach.

Afternoon snack

2 oatcakes with taramasalata

Dinner

Marie has dinner at a friend's house. She is served Thai chicken curry but forgoes the rice dish and has a larger portion of the stir-fried vegetables her friend has cooked instead. She also has a glass of wine, but refuses dessert.

Rosie

Still a teenager, Rosie, 15, lives at home, attends a day school, and is studying for her academic qualifications. Rosie's mother works full time and tries to keep plenty of healthy food in the house, but she sometimes relents and buys sweet snacks for her children. Rosie wants to be slim, and from time to time she thinks about following diets in celebrity magazines or skipping meals, but without much conviction; she manages only a day or so at most before feeling really hungry.

Rosie usually eats a low-calorie cereal and has a glass of low-calorie cranberry juice drink before she leaves for school, although she often doesn't feel like breakfast so early in the morning. At school she has a diet cola and a packet of low-fat crisps in the mid-morning break. Lunchtime is usually a salad with tuna and no dressing, or a wrap, which Rosie brings in from home. When she gets home from school in the afternoon, Rosie is always hungry and tends to have a bowl of her low-calorie cereal or some fresh fruit. If she hasn't had time to eat her lunch and is feeling really tired, she often craves something sweet. In the evening she eats whatever her mother has cooked, which might be a casserole or roast chicken with vegetables. If her parents are out, Rosie prefers a low-calorie ready-made meal for dinner.

Rosie shouldn't diet, as any marked restriction of calories at a young age will create health problems later in life; dieting is never recommended for growing teenagers, as they need nutrition, not starvation. It's also worth remembering that a consistent intake of food is especially important for young people so that their metabolism doesn't become alerted to potential 'famine'.

Rosie's mother should stick to buying healthy foods for her family, and ensure that she always has a stock of small bags of easy proteins such as nuts, seeds, and seed and cereal bars for Rosie to have as a snack with some fresh or dried fruit at school.

FOOD PLANNER FOR ROSIE

WEEKDAY 1

Breakfast
Nut-rich muesli with semi-skimmed milk for breakfast and a glass of fresh orange juice
If Rosie still wants to eat her low-calorie cereal, she can do so, but with flaked almonds sprinkled on top.

Mid-morning snack
A seed and cereal bar from a selection Rosie has bought at a healthfood store, together with an apple

Lunch
Rosie can still have a tuna salad, but with a couple of tablespoons of chick-peas and a little French dressing added to it

Afternoon snack
Natural yoghurt with some raisins and a tablespoon of mixed nuts stirred in

Dinner
Hearty fish and baby vegetable stew (p.112) cooked by Rosie's mother

WEEKDAY 2

Breakfast

Natural yoghurt with berries, pistachio nuts, and coconut flakes scattered on top, and a glass of apple juice

Mid-morning snack

An apple and 2 slices of hard cheese

Lunch

Home-made sandwich on rye bread with lots of chicken and salad and a packet of low-fat crisps

Afternoon snack

A multi-seed bagel with cream cheese and some smoked salmon

Dinner

Roast chicken (p.35) with Broccoli, cauliflower, and tomato cheese bake (p.165)

WEEKEND

Breakfast

A boiled egg and a slice of brown toast, and a small banana if Rosie is still feeling hungry

Mid-morning snack

Another seed and cereal bar from the healthfood shop with an apple

Lunch

The family eats lunch together: Grilled plaice with egg, lemon, and watercress sauce (p.120) and mashed potato and peas. Rosie's mother makes baked apples for dessert.

Afternoon snack

At her friend's house in the afternoon, Rosie has a fruit smoothie and a small bag of mixed unsalted nuts.

Dinner

Grilled lamb chops (p.51) and a green salad with some leftover Broccoli, cauliflower, and tomato cheese bake from last night

Ian I am in my mid-40s, I live in central London, and I work long hours. When working on a book, feature, or column I can work from home, but I spend at least three days a week at my office seeing clients every half hour. I always leave time for a snack in between breakfast and lunch, and again in the afternoons, as well as ensuring that I factor in a little time to eat lunch. For an instant snack I might have an apple and some raw nuts. I usually wake at 6am and exercise four times a week at 7.30am.

Rather than bulk-buying food, I prefer to buy small quantities of fresh vegetables and protein to eat within a couple of days or so. However, I always keep several cans of beans and other pulses in my store-cupboard. On holiday I tend to cook a lot more, but I still remember to prepare and reserve a little more food than I will need to eat so I can use the extra portion for a couple of snacks or as a quick meal the following day.

MY FOOD PLANNER

WEEKDAY 1

Pre-breakfast snack
On waking, I have a cup of green tea and a small bowl of natural yoghurt with toasted nuts and fresh blueberries.

Breakfast
After exercising I have an apple and a glass of protein shake (whey protein powder with soya milk).

Mid-morning snack
I drink a few cups of green or white tea throughout the morning, but mid-morning I eat a handful of walnuts and a pear.

Lunch
In the kitchen at the office I make a salad of salad leaves, canned tuna, black olives, and mixed Food Doctor seeds with a couple of oatcakes.

Afternoon snack
A small tub of natural yoghurt with some dried fruit and mixed seeds stirred into it

Dinner
Pan-roasted lamb steak (p.53) with rosemary (I omit the garlic, as I don't eat it) with steamed mangetout

WEEKEND

Breakfast

A couple of poached eggs with corn cakes, a small bowl of fruit salad, and 2 cups of green tea

Mid-morning snack

A couple of slices of hard cheese and an apple

Lunch

I'm eating out and choose an avocado and crayfish salad, followed by rib-eye steak, spinach, and a few French fries. I drink sparkling water.

Afternoon snack

A pot of natural unsweetened yoghurt with a tablespoon of mixed vanilla nuts (p.78) and blueberries on top

Dinner

A bowl of home-made vegetable soup, to which I might add chick-peas and butter beans and top with Parmesan cheese and a little truffle oil. (I make a large batch of the soup and freeze most of it in single portions.)

WEEKDAY 2

Breakfast
Natural yoghurt with oat flakes, a few raisins, and pumpkin seeds and a cup of green tea

Mid-morning snack
An apple and some walnuts

Lunch
Sliced chicken breast with salad leaves, walnuts, and cucumber and a couple of oatcakes

Afternoon snack
A couple of squares of very dark chocolate and 4–5 Brazil nuts

Late afternoon snack
I will be eating out later, so before leaving the office at around 6pm I have a few more nuts.

Dinner
Eating out in a restaurant, I avoid the breadbasket and choose gravadlax, followed by sea bass with peas and broad beans.

IAN

INDEX

Acknowledgments

Once again my grateful thanks go to Susannah Steel for her unflappable dedication, and to everyone at The Food Doctor and also at Quadrille. Special thanks to Carolyn Hughes for her delicious, innovative and practical recipes, Gabriella Le Grazie for art direction, Rob Streeter for his photography, Lucy McKelvie for cooking the dishes and to Wei Tang for styling them.